MW01251459

teach
yourself

kama sutra

teach®
yourself

kama sutra
paul jenner

For UK order enquiries: please contact Bookpoint Ltd, 130 Milton Park, Abingdon, Oxon, OX14 4SB. Telephone: +44 (0) 1235 827720. Fax: +44 (0) 1235 400454. Lines are open 09.00–17.00, Monday to Saturday, with a 24-hour message answering service. Details about our titles and how to order are available at www.teachyourself.co.uk

For USA order enquiries: please contact McGraw-Hill Customer Services, PO Box 545, Blacklick, OH 43004-0545, USA. Telephone: 1-800-722-4726. Fax: 1-614-755-5645.

For Canada order enquiries: please contact McGraw-Hill Ryerson Ltd, 300 Water St, Whitby, Ontario, L1N 9B6, Canada. Telephone: 905 430 5000. Fax: 905 430 5020.

Long renowned as the authoritative source for self-guided learning – with more than 50 million copies sold worldwide – the **teach yourself** series includes over 500 titles in the fields of languages, crafts, hobbies, business, computing and education.

British Library Cataloguing in Publication Data: a catalogue record for this title is available from the British Library.

Library of Congress Catalog Card Number: on file.

First published in UK 2007 by Hodder Education, 338 Euston Road, London, NW1 3BH.

First published in US 2007 by The McGraw-Hill Companies, Inc.

The **teach yourself** name is a registered trade mark of Hodder Headline.

Copyright © 2007 Paul Jenner

Typeset by Transet Limited, Coventry, England.
Printed in Great Britain for Hodder Education, a division of Hodder Headline, 338 Euston Road, London, NW1 3BH, by Cox & Wyman Ltd, Reading, Berkshire.

The publisher has used its best endeavours to ensure that the URLs for external websites referred to in this book are correct and active at the time of going to press. However, the publisher and the author have no responsibility for the websites and can make no guarantee that a site will remain live or that the content will remain relevant, decent or appropriate.

Hodder Headline's policy is to use papers that are natural, renewable and recyclable products and made from wood grown in sustainable forests. The logging and manufacturing processes are expected to conform to the environmental regulations of the country of origin.

Impression number   10 9 8 7 6 5 4 3 2 1
Year   2010 2009 2008 2007

contents

Dedication

This book is dedicated to the author and publisher Richard Craze, without whom I would not have written it, and who died before it was finished.

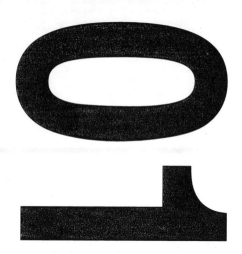

01

what this book is about

In this chapter you will learn:
- what the *Kama Sutra* is really all about
- why the *Kama Sutra* is relevant today
- how the *Kama Sutra* can improve your sex life.

Kama is the enjoyment of appropriate objects by the five senses of hearing, feeling, seeing, tasting and smelling, assisted by the mind together with the soul.

The *Kama Sutra*

Sir Richard Burton who, together with Forster Fitzgerald Arbuthnot, first brought the *Kama Sutra* to the English-speaking world, was very fond of quoting an Arab proverb:

To the pure all things are pure.

It says a lot about Burton's attitude to sex and perfectly captures that of the *Kama Sutra*, the world's oldest surviving sex manual. In the ancient Hindu culture of the time, there was no guilt about sex. When they made love, people only emulated the gods. Sex was pure.

Ever since Burton and Arbuthnot first published the *Kama Sutra* in a limited English edition more than a century ago, people have clamoured to know the ancient mysteries. And there has been no shortage of authors claiming to understand them. Today there are innumerable books, paintings, statues, cartoons, internet sites, films, videos and DVDs all purporting to reveal the secrets of the *Kama Sutra*. And most of them are fake.

Fake, that is, in the sense that they have little or nothing to do with the book called the *Kama Sutra*, compiled almost 2,000 years ago by an Indian sage known as Vatsyayana.

Teach Yourself Kama Sutra will tell you the truth. It could literally transform the whole way you think about sex and the whole way you go about it. The *Kama Sutra* is so much more than a manual of exotic sex positions. It's much richer than that.

Have a go right now

If you're anxious to get started, then here are the essential elements of *Kama Sutra*-style sex. Make love:

- with fun and games and laughter
- with, at the same time, a sense of ceremony, occasion and ritual
- in a beautiful love chamber
- surrounded by flowers, perfumes and erotic paintings
- wearing jewels and scents and decorated with body art
- with a feeling of radiance, rapture and joy
- using a wide variety of techniques and positions
- without guilt, in the knowledge that sex is the sport of the gods.

I'll be giving the full details in the rest of the book.

The world's most ancient sex secrets

The *Kama Sutra* has a strong claim to being the most ancient surviving sex manual in the world, believed to have been written in the third or fourth centuries CE. Here's a little chronology of sexual literature from the past:

- c. 2700 BCE Birth of the mythical Chinese Yellow Emperor, the central figure in Chinese sex teaching.
- c. 1250 BCE Astyanassa, the maid of Helen of Troy, writes a book of sex positions but, if true, it's now lost.
- c. 800 BCE Shvetaketu, in India, writes a *karma shastra* or 'science of love', now lost.
- c. 300 CE Vatsyayana takes the work of Shvetaketu and various other writers and compiles the *Kama Sutra*.
- c. 600 CE The *T'ung Hsüan Tzu*, a Chinese Taoist sex manual is written.
- 984 CE The *Ishimpo*, a Japanese sex manual is written by Tamba Yasuyori, but based on Chinese Taoist texts.
- c. 1000 CE The *I Hsin Fang*, a Chinese medical book is written, including extracts from earlier Chinese sex manuals.
- c. 1400 CE The *Ananga Ranga*, an Indian sex manual, is written by the poet Kalyan Mall.
- c. 1500 CE The *Perfumed Garden*, an Arabian sex manual, is written by Cheikh Nefzaoui.
- 1948 CE Kinsey publishes *Sexual Behaviour in the Human Male*.
- 1953 CE Kinsey publishes *Sexual Behaviour in the Human Female*.

Incidentally, if you think arguments about sex in the media are anything new you're wrong. The Roman poet Ovid was banished from Rome in 8 CE, partly for his *Ars Amatoria* (The Art of Love). It seems the Emperor Augustus wanted to raise the moral tone and Ovid's flippant treatment of adultery was not to his taste.

But to get back to the *Kama Sutra*, it's arguable whether India or China has the longest tradition of sex manuals. Clearly, the knowledge goes back thousands of years, and there have been tantalizing scraps of quite sophisticated sex writing recovered from Chinese tombs dating from the time of Christ. But the prize for the oldest surviving complete sex manual seems to go to the *Kama Sutra,* and that's part of its extraordinary fascination. We read it and discover that 2,000 years ago and more, people were having sex much as we do today; in some cases, better.

How the *Kama Sutra* came to be written

According to one legend, the earliest Indian text on the science of love and sex (*kama shastra*) was written by Nandi, the sacred bull, after he overheard the god Shiva making love. That must have been some session because the book ran to 1,000 chapters!

Just think how different that already is from the Western attitude to sex. A *god* making love. Enjoying sexual pleasure. Trying different positions.

> ### Have a go: write your own *Kama Sutra*
>
> On DVD/video, watch a sex scene showing something you haven't yet tried, or read about one in a book, and then, like Nandi, write a description of it. Set out all the things you'd like your partner to do to you and all the things you want to do to your partner. This is the beginning of your very own, personal *Kama Sutra*. Now do it.

Millennia after Nandi, successive generations of scholars, including a man called Shvetaketu and a whole family collectively known as 'the Babhravya', set about making the *kama shastra* more readable for ordinary people. Finally, Vatsyayana, who was a scholar probably living in the third or fourth centuries of the common era, took everything he could find from the previous thousand years or so and moulded it into a sort of 'digest' which he called the *Kama Sutra*.

Kama, as we've seen, could mean enjoyment, or pleasure, or desire. Or, as in this context, *love*. *Sutra* was a style of writing using highly condensed aphorisms. So a reasonable translation of *Kama Sutra* would be 'Aphorisms on Love'.

But that's far from the end of the story, because pithy little sayings aren't always the most unambiguous way of trying to convey information. So, for hundreds more years, yet another whole mass of scholars set about trying to explain Vatsyayana's explanation of the explanations of all the earlier ones.

Are you still with me?

One of those later scholars was a man called Yashodhara, who probably lived in the 12th century CE, and whose commentary was known as the *Jayamangala*. By popular consent, Yashodhara's explanations were the clearest and best, so Vatsyayana's *sutra* and Yashodhara's text were usually published together.

However, in fact, in his commentary, Yashodhara didn't confine himself to the *Kama Sutra*. He also drew on the *Manu Smriti* of Manu, the *Nyaya Sutra* of Gautama, the *Markendeya Purana* of Bhargava, the *Natya Shastra* by Bharata and the *Niti Shastra* of Shukra. In other words, if you were to have bought a copy of the *Kama Sutra* in Sanskrit in Bombay some time in the 19th century you'd have been getting a lot more than just the advice of Vatsyayana. You'd have been getting a whole package of stuff from different eras.

But you probably wouldn't have been able to read the Sanskrit, anyway. Which is where two Sanskrit translators, an Austro-Hungarian scholar, a British administrator in Bombay and a famous adventurer all entered the picture.

How the *Kama Sutra* came to be translated

That British administrator was Forster Fitzgerald Arbuthnot and he did, indeed, buy a copy of the *Kama Sutra* in Bombay in 1874. Arbuthnot wanted as much attention to be paid to the literature of India, where he was born, as was given to the classics of ancient Greece and Rome. And that included erotica. Especially erotica.

Arbuthnot played the role of the 'boring' civil servant, but around him he gathered some of those wonderful 19th-century eccentrics, a breed now seemingly almost extinct. Apart from two pundits (Sanskrit scholars) who translated the *Kama Sutra* into a modern Indian language, there was the Austro-Hungarian Edward Rehatsek, much given to wandering around dressed as a fakir. It was Rehatsek who took the pundits' work and translated it into English. Arbuthnot then corrected the manuscript and wrote some introductory remarks. He could have left it there and, having independent means, published it himself. But it still needed the touch of someone who was an expert in India's – indeed, virtually the world's – sexual customs and techniques. That man, an eccentric among eccentrics, one of the most extraordinary figures of his or any age, was Sir Richard Burton, explorer, anthropologist, swordsman, poet, linguist ... and sexologist. I'll be introducing you to him in Chapter 03.

The process of creating the English version of the *Kama Sutra*, therefore, was as follows:

- Various authors wrote about the 'science of love' (*kama shastra*), including Nandi (mythological), Shvetaketu and 'the Babhravya'.

- Vatsyayana took the earlier works and condensed them into some 1,250 aphorisms.

- Over the centuries that followed, various authors, most notably Yashodhara, wrote commentaries explaining the full meaning of the aphorisms.

- Arbuthnot took the aphorisms and commentaries and, aided by Bhagavanlal Indrajit and Shivaram Parashuram Bhide (the two pundits), Rehatsek and Burton, combined them into a seamless prose work that Arbuthnot and Burton jointly published as *The Kama Sutra of Vatsyayana*.

In one way it doesn't matter very much how the *Kama Sutra* as we know it in the West came into being. We can read the book, enjoy it and follow its instructions for making love. On the other hand, anyone who really wants to experience the 'erotic arts' as Vatsyayana actually intended can never be fully confident in the work as presented to us by Burton and Arbuthnot. Yashodhara, after all, was separated from Vatsyayana by hundreds of years. And for all Rehatsek's life as a 'fakir', and for all Burton's spying in the homes and harems of Karachi disguised as Mirzah Abdullah the Bushiri, they were separated from Yashodhara by a few hundred years more.

Teach Yourself Kama Sutra separates what Vatsyayana wrote from everything that came afterwards. If you want to understand the real *Kama Sutra*, if you want to make love the way it was done in India 2,000 years ago, this is the book to begin with.

But on one thing Arbuthnot and Burton couldn't be faulted. Although taking a considerable risk in Victorian Britain by publishing the book at all, they didn't suppress any of it. Their only device for 'toning down' the shock value of the text for Victorian readers was to retain the Indian word *yoni* for the vagina and the word *lingam* for the penis.

Have a go: Translating sex terms

Do you have special words for sex and the sexual parts of your body? Or do you use the dictionary words? Or don't you use any words at all? In fact, words are vital to good sex otherwise you can't tell one another what you want. There are literally hundreds of words for a *yoni*, including such quaint 19th-century terms as fireplace, inglenook, grotto, cabbage patch, cherry pie and jam pot. For a *lingam* Burton and Arbuthnot could have used lullaby (because it puts you to sleep), ladies' delight, lute, obelisk, ploughshare, pike and the member for cockshire, to list just a few. Make up your own words if you prefer, but be sure you have one for every sexy part of the body.

Now use the words to get your partner to touch you everywhere you want and how you want.

Other translations

The *Kama Sutra* published by Arbuthnot and Burton has been the standard work for more than 100 years and, unless otherwise indicated, is the version from which I quote.

Over the years since it first appeared there have been several more translations into English, of which three are currently in print. Both *The Complete Kama Sutra* translated by Alain Daniélou and *Vatsyayana Kamasutra*, translated by Wendy Doniger and Sudhir Kakar, are valuable for preserving the distinction between Vatsyayana's aphorisms and the later commentaries. On the other hand, *The Love Teachings of Kama Sutra* by Indra Sinha takes the opposite approach, rolling everything together into verses that try very much to capture the romance of the *Kama Sutra*. Full details are provided in the 'Further Reading' section at the end of the book.

So what does the *Kama Sutra* actually tell us?

As everybody knows, the *Kama Sutra* explains some fairly exotic sex techniques, especially Part Two, where Vatsyayana concentrated on foreplay and positions. But the other six sections, while dealing with such things as the 'first night', lesbian games in the harem, prostitutes and aphrodisiacs, are much more a manual of etiquette and relationships. Crucially, Vatsyayana – who was a religious student when he compiled the book – explains how sex was something sacred to the ancient Hindus. I'll have a lot more to say about that in the next chapter.

Here's a brief run-down:

• Part One: the meaning of *kama* and the life of a man-about-town in ancient India.

- Part Two: sexual techniques and positions.
- Part Three: romancing and marrying virgins.
- Part Four: the behaviour of a wife or wives, including the harem.
- Part Five: seducing other men's wives.
- Part Six: courtesans.
- Part Seven: sex toys and aphrodisiacs.

There's plenty in the *Kama Sutra* for both men and women. In that sex was considered to be a 'science', the traditionalists argued that women shouldn't read it, but Vatsyayana *wanted* women to read the *Kama Sutra*. With irrefutable logic he insisted that men couldn't have great sex with women if women didn't know how to have great sex with men. It's true that it leans towards the male viewpoint. That's how things were in those days. But there's advice here on how women can attract men … and how they can get rid of them again. There's advice on jewellery, perfume, flowers and the decoration of the 'love chamber'. And there's advice on how women can get on top.

In writing *Teach Yourself Kama Sutra* I've done my best to redress the balance between the sexes. My hope is that women and men will equally find this book enjoyable and useful.

There's controversy about the extent to which the *Kama Sutra* describes homosexual and lesbian practices. Different translators have interpreted the Sanskrit in different ways, but there's no doubt at all that the section dealing with oral sex had two men in mind more than it did a man and a woman, and in his translation, Daniélou attributes several techniques to lesbian couples. Whatever the meaning of the original text, there's plenty here that homosexual and lesbian couples can adapt.

The *Kama Sutra* and Tantra

The *Kama Sutra* is often said to be about tantric sex. However, in fact, the first complete tantric texts that have survived date from something like 300 years later. It's true that in the *Kama Sutra* sex is sacred, and tantric sex is often described as 'sacred sex', but there's an important difference: in the *Kama Sutra*, the aim of sex is always pleasure, whereas in Tantra, the aim of sex is always enlightenment.

The key difference between the *Kama Sutra* and Tantric sex (in the traditional sense) is this:

- The *Kama Sutra* is about sex for pleasure in the knowledge that sex is a sacred obligation.
- Tantric sex is about using sexual energy for spiritual advancement, whether or not pleasure is experienced.

If you'd like to know more specifically about Tantric sex you're recommended to read *Teach Yourself Tantric Sex*.

How to use this book

The next two chapters look at the sex lives of the ancient Hindus and the Victorians, into whose culture the *Kama Sutra* was hurled. These chapters are mostly for background information, although they do include some practical exercises. Skip them for now if you're anxious to get on with sex, but I recommend you return to them later for an insight into some fascinating subjects.

After that, *Teach Yourself Kama Sutra* leads you, in sequence, through every aspect of sex the ancient Indian way. If you're planning a night of love *Kama Sutra* style, then work through the chapters methodically and everything will fall into place.

Summary

- The *Kama Sutra* is the world's oldest surviving sex manual.
- It was written by Vatsyayana in India, probably in the third or fourth century CE, but based on much earlier texts, now lost.
- *Sutra* means using short, pithy sayings or aphorisms.
- Because Vatsyayana's aphorisms were sometimes difficult to understand, later writers, most famously Yashodhara, added material of their own.
- Forster Fitzgerald Arbuthnot and Sir Richard Burton published the first English translation of the *Kama Sutra*, including Yashodhara's material, in 1883.

02

the sensual world of Vatsyayana

In this chapter you will learn:
- the nature of the society in which Vatsyayana lived
- how the Hindu religion could give rise to a sex manual
- sexual attitudes in ancient India.

Man, the period of whose life is one hundred years, should practise dharma [religion], artha [the pursuit of wealth] and kama [the pursuit of pleasure] at different times and in such a manner that they may harmonize, and not clash in any way ... pleasures, being as necessary for the existence and wellbeing of the body as food, are consequently equally required ... Thus a man practising dharma, artha and kama enjoys happiness both in this world and in the world to come ... Any action which conduces to the practice of dharma, artha and kama together, or of any two, or even of one of them, should be performed ...

The *Kama Sutra*

In ancient India, the gods themselves had sex. It was a place and time of sensuality, seldom approached in the West even today. A time of pleasure, of *kama*.

Kama, as we saw in Chapter 01, could mean the enjoyment of the senses, but it was more than just that because that enjoyment had to be 'assisted by the mind together with the soul'. That's how it came about that a religious student by the name of Vatsyayana wrote the *Kama Sutra*: because sex, far from being something to feel guilty about, was an aspect of religion.

Who was Vatsyayana?

Actually, we don't know. We don't even know for sure when he lived. The best guess is in the third century of the common era, or in the fourth century, when the Gupta family began to rule an ever-growing slice of India. That certainly fits with the tone of the *Kama Sutra*. It was an era of prosperity (there were even free hospitals) when the wealthy and middle classes would have had the time for pleasure, including music, art, dancing, plays, entertainment, parties, wine and spirits (despite religious prohibitions) and, of course, sex.

Vatsyayana seems to have been a Brahman, that's to say, born into the caste of scholar-priests. His home town of Pataliputra was then one of India's greatest cities, on the banks of the Ganges. Today it's known as Patna, which is short for Pataliputra Nagara. But at some point Vatsyayana went to Benares (now known as Varanasi) as a religious student and it was there he wrote the *Kama Sutra*.

Sex and religion

To understand why a religious student would write a sex manual you have to understand the Hindu outlook of his time (very different from the Hindu outlook of today).

Hinduism covers every aspect of life and, in Vatsyayana's time, that included not only love but also sex. Note, for example, the use of the words 'mind' and 'soul' in Vatsyayana's definition of *kama*. Sensual pleasure wasn't the mere satisfaction of brute desires but was intimately connected with spiritual things. Vatsyayana was providing the 'rules'. And these weren't, by and large, rules of the Christian sort, telling people what they *couldn't* do. Quite the contrary: Vatsyayana told people which positions were the most delightful, which movements created the most excitement, which aphrodisiacs worked best and so on.

There were broadly three obligations for a Hindu:

- *Kama*, which, as we've already seen, covered desire, pleasure, love and sex.
- *Artha*, which was economic and political activity. *Artha* might seem as unlikely a religious ideal as *kama*, but the ancient Hindus took the view that when people made money for themselves they also brought benefits to the whole community.
- *Dharma*, which was religious activity.

Properly done, the three together could lead to *Moksha*, or release from the cycle of death and rebirth.

You could say that the ancient Hindus saw human sex as a kind of microcosm of the Creation, the union of Purusha (matter) with Prakriti (energy), or of Shiva, the male god, with Shakti, the goddess. One of the positions of the *Kama Sutra* is even known as *The Position Of Indrani*, the wife of one of the gods. It's unthinkable that in the Christian tradition sex positions might be named after the saints. The difference is fundamental and massive.

Where did these ideas come from? Well, in fact, from the Vedas, which were the 'Bible' of the Hindus:

- *Rig Veda* – the oldest text, written down around 1500 BCE
- *Sama Veda* – a rearrangement of the *Rig Veda*, to be sung
- *Yajur Veda* – sacrificial prayers
- *Atharva Veda* – magic, charms and incantations.

After the Vedas came:

- the *Upanishads* – over 100 texts composed between 800 BCE and 1400 CE
- followed by popular epics which illustrated the earlier teachings, particularly the *Mahabharata*, which contains within it the famous *Bhagavad Gita.*

Veda simply means 'knowledge', while *Upanishads* conveys the idea of 'learning at the feet of a master'. I say the *Rig Veda* was 'written down' rather than 'written' because Hindus believe the Vedas are *shruti*, that is to say, revealed texts that have always existed (*apaurusheya*). They weren't created by prophets but heard by *rishis* (seers) during meditation.

The Vedas explain the origin of the universe, and rather beautifully, too. They are the key to the ancient Hindu view of sex. They say there was neither what is nor what is not. That darkness was hidden in darkness. But in that infinite peace, the ONE was breathing by its own power.

The ONE, or the Divine Consciousness, which for convenience is pictured as a male god and given the name Shiva, was lonely. So Shiva created Shakti, the female. That was the moment the visible universe came into being, and everything in it works on that same principle of opposites. Male and female, positive and negative, matter and antimatter, wet and dry, hot and cold and so on.

Essentially, the whole universe is powered by Shiva and Shakti's lovemaking, which is why people must make love, too.

The *Chandogya Upanishad* explains that a woman is the 'hearth', the penis is the 'fire', that caresses are 'smoke', the vulva is the 'flame', penetration is the 'ember' and pleasure is the 'spark'. The gods 'sacrifice semen' and a child is born.

The Upanishads also tell us that the sexual organs are 'the ultimate source of pleasure', and according to the *Mahabharata*, pleasure is 'the basis of all the other aims of life'. In other words, without sex there's no *dharma*, no *artha* and no *moksha*.

Sex and ceremony

The *Kama Sutra* comes from a culture that was also very different in other ways. The ancient Hindus loved a certain theatricality. They loved rituals. In the West we've possibly never been very theatrical. In 'northern' culture, especially, we've made a cult of the 'stiff upper lip'. Understatement is one of our principal forms of humour. We love to come in from a torrential thunderstorm and announce (something like): 'It's a trifle damp out there.' And we've now done away with a lot of ritual. We don't have time for it. We always want to 'get to the point' as quickly as possible. In sex we want to go straight for the orgasm.

Vatsyayana, by contrast, was writing for people who loved embellishment, who had ceremonies for many aspects of their daily lives, who enjoyed acting a role, who loved intrigues, who loved to play games by sending messages, who used pretend quarrels as a standard feature of foreplay.

'Lad' culture in ancient India

One of the reasons for 'lad' culture was that Vatsyayana's was such a young and vibrant culture. Girls were, quite literally, displayed for marriage at puberty and the young men who chased them were probably only a few years older. So Vatsyayana was writing largely for the 'lad' culture of his time. For the more sophisticated and wealthy end of it, certainly, but for the kind of well-heeled young man who today would be getting his advice from *Esquire*, *FHM* or *GQ*. Vatsyayana's *grihastha* or house-holder would, translated into our era, spend his mornings playing the stock exchange on his laptop, his afternoons roaring around in his sports car, and his evenings throwing parties with the intention of pulling someone to spend the night with.

In fact, if you could time-travel back to ancient India you wouldn't find life too bad at all. You might even decide to stay there. Fourth-century Pataliputra, where Vatsyayana seems to have lived, might not have been 21st century London or New York, but it was a substantial town all the same. It had a nightlife. A man could have taken his girlfriends to concerts and the theatre, possibly to see *Abhijnanasakuntalam*, the masterpiece by Kalidasa, one of India's greatest poets (the dates more or less match). And in the society Vatsyayana was writing for, both men and women would have had servants to take care of just about everything. In that respect, life might have been even better than today.

Getting rid of guilt

If you feel guilty about enjoying yourself, and particularly about enjoying sex, it's hardly surprising. Western religions, in complete contrast to ancient Hinduism, see physical pleasure as a sin. And even if you're not at all religious it's hard to escape that guilty feeling. Parents live in fear of their children having sex. Children live in horror of their parents having sex. And governments pass laws about what you can and can't do, as a consenting adult, in the privacy of your own bedroom. Consider that famous advertising slogan: 'Naughty but nice'. To an ancient Hindu it would have been utterly incomprehensible. No one then would have understood how a cake could ever be 'naughty'. But, instinctively, *we* do.

If you now wish to enjoy the teachings of the *Kama Sutra* then you, too, will have to rid yourself of any sense of guilt about sex.

Have a go: entering the world of the *Kama Sutra*

The point of this exercise is to try to look at the world through the eyes of an ancient Hindu.

1 Sculptures of couples enjoying sex, known as *maithunas* or 'unions', were a normal decorative feature of Hindu temples from about 200 BCE to 300 CE. Later, whole temple facades were carved with erotic scenes. Now imagine visiting a church, perhaps your own church and finding, in addition to the usual symbols, stained glass windows depicting couples in various sexual positions. Hold on to that idea.

2 Imagine that a leading politician has appeared on TV. This is what he or she has to say: 'Sex education in our schools will now include all the positions of the *Kama Sutra*. All laws governing sexual behaviour between consenting adults are to be repealed. In addition to tea/coffee breaks, all workers are to be given time off daily for sex. Given the benefits to mental and physical health from regular sex the government will be distributing sex toys and erotica free to all households.'

3 Imagine that you're just about to have sex when the telephone rings. You answer it and instead of saying, 'Look, I'm tied up in a meeting. Can I phone you back?' you actually say, 'I'm just about to have some really lovely sex, so I'll ring you back in an hour.'

Are you ready for *kama*?

Tick the statements with which you agree.

1 I think we should eat to live and not live to eat.
2 I never masturbate.
3 When I masturbate I feel guilty afterwards.
4 I believe that sex should only happen in marriage.
5 I sometimes feel guilty after sex.
6 I feel guilty about using contraceptives.
7 I feel that sex should only be for procreation.
8 I think it's true that nice girls don't really enjoy sex.
9 I don't think people should have sex from behind because it's the way animals do it.
10 I believe that sexually transmitted diseases were sent by God to punish promiscuity.
11 I think it's polite to keep our genitals hidden from view, even while having sex.
12 I think the use of things like vibrators is unnatural and wrong.
13 I think sex shops should be banned.
14 I believe that pictures of people having sex are disgusting.

How did you score? 10–14 ticks: the *Kama Sutra* is not for you; 5–9 ticks: you have a lot of guilt about sex which you need to work on; 0–4 ticks: you're an 'ancient Hindu'.

Ancient sex secrets

In the last 60 years or so we've discovered an enormous amount about sex. We've attached electrodes to penises and put cameras up vaginas and asked people to make love in body scanners. But the ancient Hindus didn't have those things, so how could they have anything to teach us?

In fact, their scholars were just as curious as we are and, if they lacked technology, they made up for it by careful observation, practical investigation, a degree of intuition and by:

• yoga
• meditation.

Yoga was much more than a form of exercise. Going back 5,000 years, it was also a way of studying the body. Yogis can slow their heart rates, reverse the movement within their digestive tracts and achieve incredible control of their sexual organs.

Meditation, which was part of yoga, was a way of developing the mind, of concentrating its power, of focusing that power not on a distant star, as scientists might concentrate their telescopes today, but of focusing it internally. Meditation was nothing short of a scientific procedure.

The *Vedas*, the seminal books of the Hindu religion, tell us of three levels of ability:

- *Dharana* was concentrating the mind on a single thought for 12 seconds. Even this is quite difficult.
- *Dhyana* was concentrating the mind on a single thought for 12 *dharanas* – in effect meditating for nearly two and a half minutes.
- *Samadhi* or superconsciousness was the state of union with the divine energy that could be achieved by meditating for 12 *dhyanas* – almost half an hour.

Meditation could be aided by *mantras*.

Now, if you ask how the ancient Hindus could possibly know very much about sex, I might answer you with another question. How could the ancient Hindus possibly know that the universe is essentially composed of nothing more (or less) than vibrations? Indeed, Western science has now confirmed that at the atomic level matter appears as particles or waves. Hence the importance of mantras, which are words and phrases that, when pronounced correctly, *vibrate* in a special way.

Just as they discovered some of the secrets of the universe, so the ancient Hindus discovered some (but, as we'll see, not all) the secrets of sex. And as for sex between a yogi and a yogini, well, it must have been the ultimate.

Have a go: meditating on your body

Meditation is a technique that would have been used by Vatsyayana all his life. In order to learn the truth about the universe he would have been looking not outside but inside because, in Hindu belief, every person is a microcosm of the universe and in those days, the only way of understanding the macrocosm – the universe and its Creator – was to explore the microcosm which was the body.

There are essentially three stages in meditation:

- shutting off the external world
- shutting down your own thoughts
- focusing on your inner world.

Dawn and dusk are good times to meditate. Find somewhere you can sit comfortably with your back, neck and head in a straight line. It isn't essential to sit on the floor in the half lotus, but if you can manage it without strain then it helps – if your knees don't reach the floor a cushion under the rear of your buttocks will help by tilting you forwards slightly. Put your hands on your knees, palms up, with the thumb and forefinger of each hand touching to form a circle.

A well-known practice is to concentrate on an object, gazing steadily at it (*tratak*). A candle flame can be a good thing for beginners, but you could also gaze at a star or even the end of your own nose. When you can't stare any longer, close your eyes and try to visualize what you've been looking at. When the internal image fades away, look back at the real object again. As a variation, some people sit close to a blank wall and stare at that.

But we want to shut off the outer world even more completely than that. Some people like to do it physically by, for example, covering their eyes, ears, nose and mouth with their fingers (instead of putting their hands on their knees). But it's better to do it mentally if you can. To make it easier, shut doors and windows against noise and disconnect the telephone. Invite all flies to leave the room.

A powerful technique, which already existed in Vatsyayana's time, is the use of a word or phrase (mantra) whose vibrations have special qualities. Repeating the mantra over and over is known as *japa*. Every mantra has its own effect, which you won't achieve unless you're taught the special way of doing it by a guru. But, even without a guru, you can use mantras in a simpler way to help you meditate. Any short word ending in 'm' is good (Om is the best-known). While sitting as described, with your eyes closed, breathe in steadily, feeling your stomach expand. Then say your mantra, letting your breath out slowly. Just concentrate on the sound and on your own slow, steady breathing. As the 'm' hums on its way, note the vibrations through your skull, down your neck and into your chest. Eventually, you should be able to feel the vibrations reaching the ends of your fingers and the tips of your toes. You're in touch with your whole body.

Now concentrate on your heart until you can hear it beating. Once you've tuned into it, try slowing it down. See what happens when you become tense and what happens when you let all that tension go by exhaling. Next, concentrate on your genital area. Try to sense the different parts, the inner and outer labia, the clitoris and the vagina if you're a woman; the testicles, scrotum, shaft of the penis and glans if you're a man. See if you can make yourself lubricated or erect by visualizing it happening (not by thinking erotic thoughts).

Sex and the caste system

Most Westerners reject the idea that you could be trapped into a particular role in life through an accident of birth. It's against everything we believe in. However, to a Hindu, there's nothing accidental about it.

Hindus believed (and many still do) that you were given a role in society for that lifetime. (Remember that in the Hindu view there will be more lives to come.) Your task was to perform that role to the best of your ability for the good of society. By so doing you could be reincarnated in a higher role. And, of course, a prince could equally be a pauper in his next life.

There are four main castes:

- Brahmans (scholar-priests)
- Kshatriyas (kings and warriors)
- Vaishyas (farmers and merchants)
- Shudras (workers, artists and foreigners).

As a general rule, you did not socialize outside your caste, nor fall in love, nor have sex (although Vatsyayana does point out exceptions). The reason was clear: if everybody was the same, there would be no dynamism and, therefore, no universe. Above all, there could be no marriage across castes.

The *Kama Sutra* and marriage

According to the *Kama Sutra*, a man should only marry a virgin of his own caste. That was the way of 'acquiring lawful progeny and good fame'. The idea of children being of mixed caste, mixed race or mixed anything was against Hindu belief. It was that, more than anything, which could destroy that all-important diversity.

In Vatsyayana's time, marriages weren't so much *arranged* by parents as facilitated. The *Kama Sutra* tells us that: 'When a girl becomes marriageable her parents should dress her smartly, and should place her where she can be seen easily by all. [They should] show her to advantage in society, because she is a kind of merchandise.'

The *Kama Sutra* also advises that the girl should be:

- born of a highly respectable family
- possessed of wealth
- well connected

- beautiful
- of a good disposition
- with good hair, nails, teeth, ears, eyes and breasts.

Just so things aren't too one-sided, the *Kama Sutra* also adds that 'the man should, of course, also possess these qualities himself'. It may sound like the proverbial 'cattle market', but it's no different in essence from the whole idea of debutantes 'coming out', which was a standard part of the aristocratic social scene in the West until very recently.

So physical attraction, passion and lust could count just as much as other factors (but mainly on the man's part). Much harder was love, because the couple probably wouldn't have known one another in any meaningful way.

How deep is your love?

Vatsyayana says that there are ten degrees of love. Which level have you reached?

1 Love of the eye
2 Attachment of the mind
3 Constant reflection
4 Destruction of sleep
5 Emaciation of the body
6 Turning away from objects of enjoyment
7 Removal of shame
8 Madness
9 Fainting
10 Death

The *Kama Sutra* and feminism

In this age of male and female equality, you may find yourself becoming angry with some parts of the *Kama Sutra*. However, if you're a woman, don't just stop reading – in fact, the *Kama Sutra* gives you plenty of opportunity to get your revenge (as we'll see).

There's no hiding the fact that in Vatsyayana's India, women were very definitely *not* equal with men. The modern Western notion that men and women are interchangeable, both equally capable of and suited to looking after children or working on a construction site, would have been utterly incomprehensible in that culture.

In fact, even if you could time-travel to ancient India to exp
feminist thinking to women, they probably wouldn't b
interested. In the Hindu view, as we've seen, equality is death,
the end of the universe. The greater the 'inequality', on the other
hand, the greater the force of attraction between men and
women, which both sexes apparently rather enjoyed.

Have a go: being manly and womanly

Making love in accordance with the *Kama Sutra* doesn't mean
returning to the idea that women aren't equal to men. But it does
mean returning to the idea that men and women are different and
that the differences should be celebrated.

If you do believe that men and women are the same and should
be treated the same way then try to suspend that notion for a little
experiment. If you're a woman, revel in being a woman. And if
you're a man, revel in being a man. Accentuate those (undeniable)
physical differences and those (debatable) mental differences as
much as possible. Don't play them down.

- Women: put on some really feminine clothes that give plenty of
  emphasis to your curves. Accessorize with jewellery and
  perfume. Underneath, wear sexy lingerie.
- Men: wear clothes that emphasize the power of your
  shoulders. Maybe grow a moustache – a sign of virility to the
  ancient Hindus. Work out at the gym to develop your muscles.

The 64 arts

Vatsyayana was no feminist but his attitude to women was
relatively enlightened for his time. The prevailing male view, for
example, was that women couldn't study any science.
Vatsyayana, on the other hand, argued that women should
study the '64 arts' as well as his *Kama Sutra*.

In fact, 64 was a special number for the ancient Hindus and
there were two very different lists of the '64 arts'. One list
covered the sexual arts, which is the subject of this book. The
other, the one we're concerned with here, covered practical
things.

Looking down the list of the 64 'practical arts' today, many
skills remain desirable although others seem irrelevant and even
laughable. But the overwhelming feeling is awe that anybody,
man or woman, could have been an expert in them all.

...iven here in full because it provides a fascinating ...life at the time. It includes all the things connected ...ome, such as arranging flowers, cushions and carpets, ...rinks and cooking. There are games that we still play ...here are surprises such as skill with a sword and a bow ...ow. And, of course, there are all those things to do with a ...an making herself seductive, such as colouring her hair and body, creating perfumes and making jewellery. Knowledge of gymnastics was also included, which might also have been a preparation for sex.

Have a look down the list and see how many are still relevant to you today. If you were making a list of a modern 64 arts, what would you include?

1 Singing.
2 Playing musical instruments.
3 Dancing.
4 Union of dancing, singing and playing instrumental music.
5 Writing and drawing.
6 Tattooing.
7 Arraying and adorning an idol with rice and flowers.
8 Spreading and arranging beds or couches of flowers, or flowers upon the ground.
9 Colouring the teeth, garments, hair, nails and body; that, is staining, dyeing, colouring and painting them.
10 Fixing stained glass in a floor.
11 The art of making beds and spreading out carpets and cushions for reclining.
12 Playing on musical glasses filled with water.
13 Storing and accumulating water in aqueducts, cisterns and reservoirs.
14 Picture making, trimming and decorating.
15 Stringing of rosaries, necklaces, garlands and wreaths.
16 Binding of turbans and chaplets, and making crests and topknots of flowers.
17 Scenic representations. Stage playing.
18 The art of making ear ornaments.
19 The art of preparing perfumes and odours.
20 Proper disposition of jewels and decorations, and adornment in dress.
21 Magic or sorcery.
22 Quickness and dexterity in manual skill.

23 Culinary art, that is, cooking and cookery.

24 Making lemonades, sherbets, acidulated drinks, and spirituous extracts with proper flavour and colour.

25 Tailor's work and sewing.

26 Making parrots, flowers, tufts, tassels, bunches, bosses, knobs, and so on, out of yarn or thread.

28 A game that consists of repeating verses: as one person finishes, another person has to commence at once, repeating another verse, beginning with the same letter with which the last speaker's verse ended. Whoever fails to repeat is considered to have lost and to be subject to pay a forfeit or stake of some kind.

29 The art of mimicry or imitation.

30 Reading, including chanting and intoning.

31 Study of sentences difficult to pronounce. It is played as a game, chiefly by women and children, and consists of a difficult sentence being given; and when it is repeated quickly, the words are often transposed or badly pronounced.

32 Practise with the sword, single-stick, quarterstaff and bow and arrow.

33 Drawing inferences, reasoning or inferring.

34 Carpentry, or the work of a carpenter.

35 Architecture, or the art of building.

36 Knowledge about gold and silver coins, jewels and gems.

37 Chemistry and mineralogy.

38 Colouring jewels, gems and beads.

39 Knowledge of mines and quarries.

40 Gardening: knowledge of treating the diseases of trees and plants, of nourishing them and determining their ages.

41 The arts of cockfighting, quail fighting and ram fighting.

42 The art of teaching parrots and starlings to speak.

43 The art of applying perfumed ointments to the body, and of dressing the hair with unguents and perfumes and braiding it.

44 The art of understanding writing in cipher and the writing of words in a peculiar way.

45 The art of speaking by changing the forms of words. It is of various kinds. Some speak by changing the beginning and end of words, others by adding unnecessary letters between every syllable of a word, and so on.

46 Knowledge of languages and of the vernacular dialects.

47 The art of making flower carriages.

48 The art of framing mystical diagrams, of addressing spells and charms, and binding armlets.

49 Mental exercises, such as completing stanzas or verses on receiving a part of them; or supplying one, two or three lines when the remaining lines are given indiscriminately from different verses, so as to make the whole an entire verse with regard to its meaning; or arranging the words of a verse written irregularly by separating the words from the consonants, or leaving them out altogether; or putting into verse or prose sentences represented by signs or symbols. There are many other such exercises.

50 Composing poems.

51 Knowledge of dictionaries and vocabularies.

52 Knowledge of ways of changing and disguising a person's appearance.

53 Knowledge of the art of changing the appearance of things, such as making cotton to appear as silk, coarse and common things to appear as fine and good.

54 Various ways of gambling.

55 The art of obtaining possession of the property of others by means of mantras or incantations.

56 Skill in youthful sports.

57 Knowledge of the rules of society, and of how to pay respects and compliments to others.

58 Knowledge of the art of war: arms, armies, and so on.

59 Knowledge of gymnastics.

60 The art of knowing the character of a man from his features.

61 Knowledge of scanning or constructing verses.

62 Arithmetical recreations.

63 Making artificial flowers.

64 Making figures and images in clay.

Prostitution

As we've seen, a couple might have married because a man was physically attracted to the girl who was 'merchandise', but she would usually have been little more than a child with no experience of sex or anything else. In fact, she was likely to be so inexperienced that the *Kama Sutra* advises the man to wait until 'the night of the tenth day' after the marriage to attempt intercourse. Such relationships could grow into love, of course, but if they didn't, there was no easy escape for a woman. For a man, on the other hand, there were always the 'public women'.

There was no stigma attached to prostitution in Vatsyayana's time. Since sex itself was sacred, and since making money was revered as *artha*, so putting the two things together was perfectly in keeping with the ancient Hindu moral and religious outlook. Courtesans, as opposed to 'water carriers' who might be forced into sex, were highly respected. Those who had mastered the 64 arts (both sets, presumably) were known as *ganikas* and, the *Kama Sutra* tells us, would even receive 'a seat of honour' wherever men were gathered.

However, the *Kama Sutra* mostly advises about – as we might say nowadays – kept women. That's to say, there was a relationship of sorts. For the woman it was based on money, but for the man there would have been a genuine attraction and maybe even love.

Goodbye to paradise

The Hindu culture of ancient India was a sexual paradise that lasted for thousands of years. It reached its climax with the beautiful and fabulously erotic sculptures on the temples of the Chandella kings at Khajuraho in Madhya Pradesh. But even as the stonemasons were putting the finishing touches to the *yonis* and *lingams* and entwined couples, so people with a very different view were gathering their armies on India's frontiers.

Sex and the Muslim invasions

For many Hindus, the good sex life started to unravel in the 11th century with the first of the Muslim invasions. Geography dictated that they came from the north and west which is why, today, the area that's now Pakistan is strongly Muslim whereas the south of India remains almost entirely Hindu.

Muslim ideas were very different from Hindu ideas. Overt sensuality became wrong. Everybody had to be covered to prevent sexual temptation. Women who had sometimes gone bare-breasted were shrouded from head to foot and shut away. So, there was great change. Sex was confined to marriage. Sometimes special taxes were imposed on non-Muslims, forcing the Hindus to convert. The age of the *Kama Sutra* was over.

Sex and the British invasion

The situation got even worse when the British arrived. The initial liaison that had begun with trade culminated in 1818 in a settlement that gave Britain's East India Company control of much of India.

Those Indians who wanted to prosper under British rule adopted British ways. Queen Victoria was born one year after the settlement, became Queen of Great Britain and Ireland in 1837 and was proclaimed Empress of India in 1876. Unfortunately for their sex lives, the Anglicized Indians were buying into a culture that thought sex was dirty rather than beautiful – the Victorian culture. In the next chapter we'll see how the Victorians had sex.

Summary

- The ancient Hindus believed that sex (*kama*) was a sacred part of their religion.
- Although certain sexual practices were forbidden, there was no guilt about *kama*.
- If you want to enjoy *kama* you, too, must rid yourself of any guilt about sex.
- The ancient Hindus used yoga and meditation to intuit all kinds of things that Western science has now proven to be true.
- Yoga and meditation can be used to discover and control your own body.
- The ancient Hindus believed that opposite forces provided the universe with its energy.
- They therefore believed, that men and women should be as opposite as possible.
- Prostitution was sacred in ancient India.
- The relatively free sexual attitudes of the ancient Hindus became more restrictive under Muslim rule and more restrictive again under British rule – the world of the *Kama Sutra* seemed to be over.

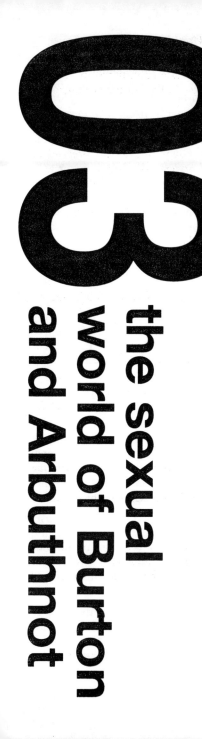

03

the sexual world of Burton and Arbuthnot

In this chapter you will learn:
- 19th-century attitudes to sex
- why Burton and Arbuthnot wanted to change those attitudes
- Victorian sex practices.

Vatsyayana says that the man should begin to win her over, and to create confidence in her, but should abstain at first from sexual pleasures. Women being of a tender nature, want tender beginnings, and when they are forcibly approached by men with whom they are but slightly acquainted, they sometimes suddenly become haters of sexual connection ...

The *Kama Sutra* on marriage:

Many a life has been wasted and the best feelings of a young woman outraged by the rough exercise of what truly become the husband's 'rights', and all the innate delicate sentiments and illusions of the virgin bride are ruthlessly trampled on when the curtains close around the couch on what is vulgarly called the 'first night'...

Forster Fitzgerald Arbuthnot,
co-translator of the *Kama Sutra*

If Vatsyayana could have been transported from fourth-century Benares to 19th century London he would have found many aspects of life surprisingly familiar. For a start, and contrary to popular belief, the Victorians were as fun loving as the ancient Hindus. They were, after all, the first members of an industrial society to enjoy leisure time and the first to take holidays.

Both societies routinely indulged in drugs. While the Indians had their betel and cannabis, the Victorians had their laudanum, a mixture of opium and alcohol, which was prescribed as a painkiller in a wide range of conditions from a simple headache to tuberculosis. Being cheaper than gin it was extremely popular. Cocaine was also easily available and in 1863 a wine laced with cocaine and known as Vin Mariani was successfully launched. Apparently, even Queen Victoria enjoyed it.

Vatsyayana would have been quite at ease with the British caste system which was known as 'class'. As a foreigner he would have expected to be received as a Shudra, the lowest of the four main Hindu castes, and would have perfectly understood that he could never be a member of the aristocracy, just as he could never be a Kshatriya back home.

Vatsyayana wouldn't have been surprised that there were prostitutes but he would have been puzzled by the way they were treated. With the exception of a few famous 'courtesans' they would have been relegated to the back streets, uneducated in the 64 arts and held in contempt.

Estimates of the number of prostitutes who worked in London in the latter part of the 19th century vary considerably, but around 50,000 is probably about right. Many women prostituted themselves only occasionally, or during a short difficult period, just to get by. But generally they operated in a low-key way. There were only a few brothels, like that run by Mary Jeffries in the 1870s which was equipped with a torture chamber for indulging the masochistic fantasies of the aristocracy. Knowing all about the relationship between pain and pleasure, Vatsyayana would only have been surprised at the extremes some Victorians were going to.

He would have been astonished that there were hardly any sex manuals. But he would have been able to buy books of erotic stories such as *Lady Pokingham*, *They All Do It* and *My Secret Life*, by 'Walter', which recounted sex with 1,000 women. He wouldn't have been able to see any erotic sculptures or erotic stained-glass windows at any churches but he would have been able to obtain magic lantern slides, daguerreotypes and photographs of naked women. One of the most successful pornographic photographers of the day was Henry Hayler who had a studio in Pimlico. Lesbian scenes were particularly popular.

Did Victorians know about the clitoris?

In a libel action in 1918 one witness gave evidence that a clitoris 'was a superficial organ that, when unduly excited or overdeveloped, possessed the most dreadful influence on any woman, that she would do the most extraordinary things'. Another witness, a Dr Cooke, announced that clitoris was a word 'nobody but a medical man or people interested in that kind of thing would understand'.

But 'Walter', the author of *My Secret Life*, published in 11 volumes towards the end of the Victorian era, understood the word very well. His romp contains the word 'clitoris' 434 times. There were also 227 references to 'gamahuche', which means fellatio or cunnilingus. 'Walter' is believed to have been Henry Spencer Ashbee, a friend of both Burton and Arbuthnot.

Vatsyayana would have had little problem with the position of married women in Victorian Britain. Just as in ancient India, their role was confined to the home. There they had a certain power but they were expected to be humble with regard to their husbands. In other words, just as in the *Kama Sutra*, they were to treat men like gods.

Where our Hindu time-traveller would have been utterly perplexed would have been a man's treatment of his wife in bed. Far from them running through a variety of positions in which she boldly displayed herself for his pleasure, he would have been furtively sliding under heavy sheets to discharge his sexual tension in less time than an ancient Hindu spent on the first kiss.

Obviously, attitudes didn't remain the same throughout the 60 or so years of the Victorian era and, in fact, there were two quite permissive decades, the 1860s and the 1890s. But in general the Victorians were reformers and modernizers and that applied to sex as much as anything else. As they saw it, sex was an animal thing which sophisticated people only used for procreation.

Victorian women, if they were well-educated and modern, were therefore generally passive in sex and men were usually either apologetic or aggressive. A story, an urban myth of the time if you like, is of a self-chloroformed bride on her wedding night with a note pinned to her pillow saying: 'Mama says you're to do what you like.'

Far from being delighted at the possibility of their wives reading the *Kama Sutra* and becoming enthusiastic about sex, most Victorian husbands would have been appalled. Nice women didn't behave like that and, above all, Victorian men wanted nice women.

Sir Richard Burton

Sir Richard Burton was one of the most extraordinary men to bestride the Victorian age. He was a sexologist before sexologists had ever been invented. Everywhere he went in the world he enquired into sexual behaviour and, certainly for about the first 20 years of his adult life, his researches included plenty of personal experience. Apart from his role in bringing the *Kama Sutra* to Britain, Burton also had a hand in the translation of another classic Indian erotic text, the 14th or 16th-century CE *Ananga Ranga* by the poet Kalyan Mall. He translated the Arabian sex manual *The Perfumed Garden* of Sheikh Nefzaoui from a French edition (and later revised it from an Arabic text). He translated the *Arabian Nights*. He translated the *Priapeia*, a compilation of erotic verse by various Roman poets. Oh yes, and he also *almost* discovered the source of the Nile.

Burton was a Victorian fictional hero come to life. No Sherlock Holmes could possibly compete. To begin with, he was a man of startling physical appearance. Tall, with muscular shoulders and chest he was, among other things, an expert swordsman. A portrait of Burton, aged around 40, painted by his friend Louis Desanges, shows him with intense, brooding eyes, powerful features and a flamboyant and dangerous-looking moustache which hung down from his chin on each side.

If he was physically imposing, he was intellectually terrifying. He could speak more than a score of languages fluently and his writings are full of the sort of references that, although easy in the computer age, required an encyclopaedia of a brain in his era. He was also a poet, a scientist and an outstanding anthropologist.

There isn't space to go into all of Burton's adventures in this book but it's clear that, serving in India around the middle of the 19th century, he knew the country's sexual customs at first hand. He fell in and out of love regularly, with native women as well as white, his mistresses including a dancer called Núr Ján (Radiant Light). Around 1847–48 he jotted down a poem called *Past Loves* in which he said he 'flirted with about a mile/of Whites, Browns and Reds/Yellows and browns of every race/Tawny Body and sooty face/full bred and (sometimes) half bred …'

With his language skills and high-cheekboned swarthy appearance he often went 'under cover'. In disguise he visited the brothels of Karachi (now in Pakistan, of course), penetrated harems while pretending to be a merchant in muslins and jewellery, stayed at inns where hemp and opium were available (and happily used both) and was even once venerated as a holy man. So his translation of the *Kama Sutra* was infused with an intimate knowledge of Hindu culture as well as its sexual techniques.

Later expeditions brought him into contact with the sexual world of the Middle East (he visited Mecca and Medina in disguise, having had himself circumcised as a precaution) and Africa.

His sexual adventures (but not his others) came to an end when he was 40, in 1861 when he married the aristocratic Isabel Arundell.

Isabel Arundell

In one way it hardly seemed a good match. Richard was a sort of cross between Kinsey, Ranulph Fiennes and Mick Jagger while Isabel was highly religious and at nearly 30 years old almost certainly still a virgin. His biographers veer between those who say his marriage was a disaster and those who say it was a great passion.

New evidence supports the latter group. For her it was a great passion from the very beginning and, for him, it became so. Isabel's Victorian spinsterhood till age 29 wasn't a sign of frigidity but the reverse. As for any Victorian woman of her class, sex was unthinkable outside marriage. She'd been 'saving herself' ever since setting eyes, ten years earlier on the ramparts in Boulogne, on a man with 'black flashing eyes' that, she wrote, 'pierced one through and through'. Once she learned his name there was no escape for her. Five years earlier a gypsy had foretold that she would marry a man with the name of Burton. Perhaps it was destiny or, as the Arabs say, kismet.

As for Burton, he didn't yet know this. Four years after that first meeting with Isabel he had to abandon an expedition following a diagnosis of syphilis. It wasn't for another year that he proposed. Yet another five years passed before they could marry, partly because of Richard's expeditions but largely because of the opposition of Isabel's mother.

Just before the gypsy's prediction finally came true, Isabel compiled her *Rules for my Guidance as a Wife*, and they're rather intriguing in two ways. Firstly, although there were only 17 of them, rather than the Kama Sutra's 64, they echoed Vatsyayana's essential arts in several ways. The fourth rule, for example, was this:

- Improve and educate yourself in every way, that you may enter into his pursuits and keep pace with the times, that he may not weary of you.

More significantly, there was something very (ancient) Hindu about them.

- … let him find in the wife what he and many other men fancy is only to be found in a mistress, that he may seek nothing out of his home.
- Do not try to hide your affection for him, but let him see and feel it in every action … keep up the honeymoon romance, whether at home or in the desert.

Like any Hindu wife she vowed to treat him as a god. And this is what she did.

In reality, it doesn't take very long to learn the basics of sex, even as a 29 year-old virgin. And Burton would have had the capacity to be one of the finest teachers in the world. 'Women all the world over,' he wrote in his *Terminal Essay* to the *Arabian Nights*, 'are what men make them ...'. No doubt he made her the lover he wanted. For Isabel's part, it only required the right mental attitude, and it would seem she had that. 'I was,' she wrote in her diary, 'born for love.'

Have a go: write some rules

Set out your own rules of behaviour for yourself. You don't necessarily have to show them to anybody and you probably won't always abide by them, but at least you'll be setting down an ideal of how you'd like to behave. And it's a useful exercise for trying to understand your own feelings.

While you're at it, write down all the good things about your partner. Make a note of the sacrifices made, the problems overcome, the noble deeds ...

When you've had a row, read it all through.

Forster Fitzgerald Arbuthnot

Arbuthnot and Burton had a lot in common. At 12 years younger than Burton, with short wavy hair but the usual long Victorian beard, he was actually born in India and spent most of his working life there until retiring to Guildford and marriage in 1879. The two had met in 1854, when Burton was in Bombay getting ready for his Somalia expedition. The two hit it off and Burton took to calling him 'Bunny'. It seems to have been 'Bunny' rather than Burton who had the idea of translating and publishing Indian erotica. Up until then, Burton's prolific output of more than a score of books had been concerned largely with travel and anthropology.

The *Ananga Ranga*

Before collaborating on the *Kama Sutra*, Burton and Arbuthnot had worked together on a more recent Indian sex manual, the

Ananga Ranga, written by a poet called Kalyan Mall, probably in the 14th or 15th centuries.

Given that Britain had recently passed the Obscene Publications Act the two men were running a serious risk. With their interest in India the two could, for example, have published the Vedas or the Upanishads without any danger at all. But they had strong and rather similar motives for promoting sex books.

In a letter to Henry Spencer Ashbee, Arbuthnot explained: 'Many a life has been wasted and the best feelings of a young woman outraged by the rough exercise of what truly become the husband's "rights"...' Ignorance of sex, he believed, 'has unfortunately wrecked many a man and many a woman.'

Burton gave his outlook in his *Terminal Essay* to the *Arabian Nights*: 'Moslems and Easterns in general study and intelligently study the art and mystery of satisfying the physical woman,' he wrote. Their youngsters, he explained with approval, attended sex courses that lasted anything from a few days to a year. By contrast, it was 'said abroad that the English have the finest women in Europe and least know how to use them'.

There seems to have been more than a touch of personal bitterness in the feelings of both men.

The *Ananga Ranga* also had the chance of making serious money. Erotica aside, very few books that had anything at all to say about sex were available in Victorian Britain. A lucky couple might be able to get hold of *Kalogynomia: or the Laws of Female Beauty* by Dr T. Bell, printed in 1821, or *Every Woman's Book* by Dr Waters published in 1826, or *The Elements of Social Science of Physical, Sexual and Natural Religion,* by a 'Doctor of Medicine' published three years before the *Kama Sutra* in 1880. But in general, sex was neither written about nor, in polite society, talked about.

However, it was not to be a publishing success at first. In 1873, after a few proof copies were run off, the printer took fright and it wasn't finally published until 1885.

Meanwhile, both men had noted the *Ananga Ranga's* intriguing references to a sage called 'Vatsya'. The search was on for India's ancient sex secrets.

Publishing the *Kama Sutra*

Returning to India from 'home' leave in 1874, Arbuthnot immediately began searching for copies of the *Kama Sutra*. Eventually he found one in Bombay, but it was considered to be 'defective' in some way, presumably because parts were missing. His pundits (Sanskrit scholars) then wrote to the great libraries in Benares, Calcutta and Jeypoor to ask for copies to be made. All four versions were then compared and a master version finally compiled.

At some point the decision was taken to present Vatsyayana's aphorisms and Yashodhara's commentary on them (the *Jayamangala*) as a continuous work of prose. In other words, the distinction between what Vatsyayana originally wrote and what Yashodhara wrote the best part of a thousand years later was completely lost. What's more, when things weren't clear, Burton and Arbuthnot also drew on other sex manuals and commentaries.

Arbuthnot would immediately have seen that, as a publishing venture, the *Kama Sutra* had one great advantage over the *Ananga Ranga*. Whereas the latter confined itself entirely to sex, the *Kama Sutra* covered every aspect of social conduct in respect of sex, love and marriage. It could therefore far more easily be passed off as a work of anthropological scholarship in order to get round the Obscene Publications Act of 1857.

Arguably, the Act didn't cover material printed for private circulation, so as an extra precaution the two men formed the Kama Shastra Society of Benares and London, which would only make the book available to private subscribers. The two men also concealed their identities – although not very well.

Unfortunately, no records seem to exist regarding the early sales of the *Kama Sutra* following its publication in 1883. Burton died seven years later at the age of 69.

The Victorians and sex

Of course the Victorians had sex. Many Victorian couples no doubt had attitudes no different from those of today. At one end of the spectrum were those who ran and used brothels, wrote erotic novels, produced pornographic photographs and practised free love. In the middle were the vast majority of couples. And at the opposite end of the spectrum were those who ran the Social Purity campaign, arguing that civilization should transcend 'animal' instincts.

But, guilt aside, the big difference between Victorian sex and modern sex was contraception. Victorian sex carried with it a high risk of pregnancy. And pregnancy carried with it a high risk of death as well as, if outside marriage, exclusion from 'polite society'. Understandably, women weren't always keen on having a lot of sex, even if they had no hang-ups about its 'animal' nature.

In fact, contraceptives of a sort were available. When Isabel and Richard Burton married they could have used, if they wanted, the vulcanized rubber condom that Goodyear and Hancock put into production in 1844. But sensitive it was not. It was about as thick as a pair of rubber gloves and after each use had to be washed and carefully returned to its box. Curiously enough, the first thinner latex condoms made their appearance around the time the *Kama Sutra* was published in Britain. But they didn't really catch on until the 1930s. Why? Because churches said contraception was immoral and governments said it was illegal.

In the USA, the Comstock Law of 1873 prohibited the advertising of any sort of birth control and allowed the postal service to confiscate condoms and birth control literature sent through the mail, something that was still going on right up to the 1940s. Meanwhile, in the UK the attitude was more or less the same and in 1877 Annie Besant and Charles Bradlaugh were actually put on trial for publishing a book on methods of birth control. All the Christian denominations were unanimous in condemning birth control until the Church of England broke ranks by allowing contraception for married couples in 1930. In the Victorian era, then, abstinence seemed to be the only solution if you didn't want a large family.

Victorian sexual practices

Curiously, it was precisely this lack of contraception that led many well-educated Victorians towards sexual experimentation. They wanted to find a way of having sex without the risk of pregnancy.

One solution that worked quite well was 'invented' by a man called John Humphrey Noyes. In a pamphlet called *Male Continence*, Noyes described how his wife became pregnant five times in six years (four of the babies dying) and how he became determined to find a way of enjoying sex without 'procreation'.

He likened sex for a man to a 'stream in three conditions':

- a fall
- a course of rapids above the fall
- still water above the rapids.

Noyes' technique was to remain in 'the region of easy rowing'. That's to say, a man could approach ejaculation, but never so closely as to risk 'going over' the falls.

Noyes was obviously more than an ancient Hindu in spirit, because he decided not to confine his discovery to himself and his wife. Instead, he went on to establish the 'utopian' Oneida Community in New York in 1848, which practised 'complex marriage' or, as we'd say nowadays, free love. Members of the community had, on average, about three different partners a week and, although there were some pregnancies, they were far below the normal level.

Have a go: male continence

Male continence is similar to the technique nowadays known as stop/go. Essentially, as soon as a man starts to feel himself getting too excited he ceases all stimulation until the excitement has faded sufficiently for him to resume.

A word of warning first of all. Do not use *male continence* for birth control. It works better than nothing at all but it's far from foolproof. Some sperm will always leak out, no matter how good your technique. Use it instead as a way of prolonging intercourse.

Practise, first of all, during masturbation. Don't try with your partner until you've gained a good measure of control. You need to be able to identify the point at which, in Noyes' analogy, your boat will inevitably go over the falls. The so-called 'point of no return'. To complicate matters, there can be a delay of up to three seconds between reaching the point and actually ejaculating.

Sometimes you will go 'over the falls' by mistake. Don't worry about it. Just enjoy it. Remember, Noyes recommended staying well back in the 'still water' where the pleasure is less intense but control far easier to achieve.

It's largely a mental technique. There's a strong compulsion to go over those falls but you have to resist it.

With your partner you can decide to ejaculate eventually since you'll be using effective contraception. Or you can decide to follow Noyes' formula to the letter. Some men do, because it means they can have sex again all the sooner. If you are going to try that, discuss it with your partner first. She may miss your orgasm.

Noyes' technique can be taken much further, giving men orgasm without ejaculation (see Chapter 11).

Karezza

The Oneida Community used male continence as a way of pursuing *Kama Sutra*-type sexual pleasure without the risk of pregnancy. Almost half a century later, towards the end of the Victorian era, a woman called Alice Bunker Stockham devised a similar technique but, in her case, it was for a different reason. She wanted to make sex something more spiritual than physical. She called it *Karezza*.

Stockham was born into a Quaker family on the American frontier in 1833, where her outlook may well have been influenced by the native Americans among whom she lived. She went on to become only the fifth woman doctor in the USA and held modern views on the importance of a high-fibre diet, exercise during pregnancy, the role of the mind in illness and – one of her favourite subjects – the danger of corsets.

Stockham travelled to India and what she learned there resulted in her book *Karezza*, a name she created from the Italian word *carezza*, meaning 'caress'. It's a fairly apt title because she recommended that during intercourse couples do just that and little more.

The Hindu influence on her devout Christianity is clear in sentences like these:

- 'He is a spiritual parent who has learned to drink from the well of truth, and from the deep resources of his being, has discovered the secret powers of life.'

- 'In the physical union of male and female there may be a soul communion giving not only supreme happiness, but in turn [leading] to soul growth and development.'

But she was at odds with Hinduism in her feminist insistence that women and men were equal: 'The knowledge of the living, spiritual truth that man has no separate existence from God, is the most potent factor in breaking down all supposed inequalities between the sexes.'

Initially, Stockham's method, like Noyes', was for the man to avoid ejaculating but for his partner to have as many orgasms as she could manage. Later, however, Stockham revised her method to say that neither would have an orgasm. Stockham's reasoning was that if avoiding orgasm heightened spiritual experience then the woman should be able to share that equally with the man.

Have a go: *Karezza*

Decide beforehand which form of Karezza you're going to go for. In other words, is it only the man who is going to avoid orgasm or is it both of you? I'd suggest both of you, firstly because it's going to be easier and secondly because for the woman to deliberately avoid orgasm is going to be something new.

The first thing you have to do in *Karezza* is make a sort of spiritual dedication. You might, for example, exchange love letters or you might do something more religious.

Next, spend some quiet time together to get in the right frame of mind. Stockham suggested reading poetry to one another, but you could also share wine, light candles and incense and listen to music.

When you begin to make love, do it slowly and gently. Avoid thrusting. Just relax and wallow in the sense of being together. Keep this going for at least an hour. That, according to Stockham, was the minimum time necessary to experience the feeling of 'total union' and 'holy love'. Sometimes she saw lights glowing.

How was it possible for a man to maintain an erection so long with so little stimulation? The answer is that while Stockham said couples could practise *Karezza* as often as they liked, her recommendation was to leave 'an interval of two to four weeks' between lovemaking sessions. 'And many find that even three to four months afford greater impetus,' she concluded.

So hers wasn't so very different from the Victorian idea of sex after all.

Marie Stopes

Britain's equivalent to Alice Bunker Stockham was Marie Stopes. Stopes was a remarkable woman who fought the Establishment on several fronts, not least by setting up the birth-control clinics that still bear her name. Her mother was the first woman in Scotland to obtain a university certificate and Marie became Britain's youngest doctor of science in 1905. After several love affairs she married a man called Reginald Gates, but the marriage was a disaster and was annulled five years later on the grounds of non-consummation. That experience spurred her to write one of the most beautiful and lyrical 'sex manuals' ever published, under the title *Married Love*. First brought out in 1918, it sold 2,000 copies within a fortnight, and for those who believe no one in Britain knew about the clitoris until 1960 the book gives a detailed description. Theoretically, the Victorian era was over but in Britain the book caused outrage and in America it was banned as obscene.

It's important to remember that by the standards of the time, Stopes was an enthusiast for sex. A dangerous woman. Yet, nowadays, her ideas seem quaint. From questioning her female patients as to what men then called 'contrariness' she drew up her 'law of Periodicity of Recurrence of desire'. She concluded that the average woman felt two 'wave-crests' of desire in each monthly cycle, spaced roughly two weeks apart. The first occurred two to three days before menstruation and the second, weaker crest came eight to nine days after the end of menstruation. Unfortunately, the first wave crest lasted only three days down to a 'few hours, or even less'. The second was even shorter. The comical image springs to mind of husbands sprinting up the stairs only to be told: 'Sorry, darling, you missed it again.'

Stopes wasn't quite prepared for some of her own findings. 'There are a very few women,' she wrote, 'who seem to be really a little abnormal, who feel the strongest desire actually during the menstrual flow.' Nowadays this is common knowledge, but at the time it was an embarrassing concept.

Through her work Stopes heard plenty of Victorian-style horror stories. There were couples who didn't know how to have sex at all. There was the husband who was so frightened when his wife once had an orgasm that he thought she'd had a fit. But, most of all, there were women who just never orgasmed – about 70 to 80 per cent of her clients, Stopes estimated.

Significantly, Stopes was opposed to *coitus interruptus* (the man withdrawing and ejaculating outside the vagina). She proclaimed this Victorian birth control method bad for women because, among other things, it prevented them absorbing a man's 'secretions'. Her formula for great sex was therefore to have a little orgy for three or four days then take ten days off. That way, a man's 'vital energy and nerve-force', as well as his 'precious chemical substances', could be retained for other 'creative' things the rest of the time. That was precisely what many Eastern sexual philosophies also believed.

Summary

- There are surprising similarities between the culture of ancient India and Victorian culture.
- Some Victorians did know about the clitoris, but Victorian women were generally passive in bed.
- Sir Richard Burton's sexual experiences in India and elsewhere ideally suited him for the role of commentating on and publishing the *Kama Sutra*, together with Forster Fitzgerald Arbuthnot.
- Before working together on the *Kama Sutra*, Burton and Arbuthnot tried to publish the *Ananga Ranga*, another Indian sex manual, but their printer refused.
- The promotion of contraception was actually illegal in both Britain and the USA at the time.
- Victorian techniques to avoid pregnancy included male continence and *Karezza*.
- In her clinics, Marie Stopes found that between 70 and 80 per cent of women never experienced orgasm.

04

preparing yourself for kama

When the wife wants to approach her husband in private, her dress should consist of many ornaments, various kinds of flowers, and a cloth decorated with different colours, and some sweet-smelling ointments or unguents.

Now, the householder... should wash his teeth, apply a limited quantity of ointments and perfumes to his body, put some ornaments on his person and collyrium on his eyelids and below his eyes, colour his lips with alacktaka and look at himself in the glass ...

The *Kama Sutra*

In the *Kama Sutra*, making love wasn't something you did because you were going to bed anyway. Sex was a celebration, a party, a rite, a ritual and a religious ceremony all rolled into one.

Nowadays, in the West, most of us have rituals only for very significant occasions, such as baptism, marriage and death. The ancient Hindus had these as well, of course, but they also had rituals concerning many aspects of their daily lives. Just taking a bath had to be done in a particular way. You could say that always adding the same fragrant oil to your bath is a private ritual, or always carving the Sunday roast at the table. But these are nothing compared with the elaborate rules the ancient Hindus (and many people in the East even today) observed. And, of course, the same applied to sex.

Kama cosmetics

In the West, men are only just starting to use cosmetics again. But at various times in the past it's been just as normal for men to apply a little 'paint' as for women. In Vatsyayana's day, men used both lipstick and eyeliner. Unfortunately, Vatsyayana didn't describe the cosmetics a woman should use, but they certainly would have included those things. According to the *Kama Sutra* our man-about-town should, every day:

• take a bath
• clean his teeth
• apply ointments and perfumes
• put collyrium on his eyelids and below his eyes
• put *alacktaka* on his lips
• eat betel leaves to make his mouth fragrant
• put on ornaments.

He should also:

- anoint his body with oil every other day
- use a lathering substance every three days
- shave his head and face every four days
- shave the rest of the body every five to ten days.

As we'll see, the *Kama Sutra* recommends spending a lot of time kissing, so lovers in Vatsyayana's time would have been just as concerned with bad breath as we are today. In fact, the ancient Hindus had toothpaste. It was made of cardamom, cinnamon, honey and black pepper together with sandalwood powder which had been mixed with – wait for it – cow's urine. So it should certainly have given as much tingle as a modern toothpaste. It was applied with a stick, not a brush.

The equivalent of mouthwash was betel, but in addition to making the mouth fragrant, betel leaves were also used as a drug. I'll have more to say about that in the next chapter.

The final touch was provided by a kind of lipstick called *alacktaka*. A ball of red lacquer would first be rubbed over the lips to colour them and then fixed by rubbing a ball of beeswax on top, rather like a modern lip gloss.

Have a go

- Teeth: use an electric toothbrush, floss daily and visit the dental hygienist at least twice a year.
- Eyes: collyrium was what we'd now call kohl. Women already use eye make-up, but if you're a man, why not try eye liner and see what it does for you?

Shaving and waxing

A clear view of the vulva is as exciting to a man today as it ever was to an ancient Hindu. So try surprising your man. Or let him trim your locks to his own personal taste as a little bit of love play.

Tip

- Women: a woman's electric razor or man's beard trimmer work perfectly well, but for a really smooth job you may prefer a professional waxing. The general idea is to remove all the hair from around the outer vaginal lips, leaving just a little tuft above the clitoris. If you have fairly thick hair on the mons (the fleshy little mound just below your navel) you may be able to do something interesting with it, like trim it into a V-shape. Some women remove everything.

- Men: it's only polite to trim pubic hair to make sure it doesn't get in the way during oral sex. And while you're at it why not – if only for a laugh – go the whole hog. At the very least it will make you seem quite a bit longer, which is always good for self-confidence.

Ornaments, jewellery and clothing

Whenever you see illustrations of the *Kama Sutra*, whether modern or antique, lovers are seldom entirely naked. The man is always wearing, at the very least, some sort of hat or turban and maybe a short tunic or even a cloak. The woman usually has her hair free but often has something around her shoulders or some kind of band around her waist. And both will be covered in jewellery. As the *Kama Sutra* emphasizes, a woman who wants to make love should wear 'many ornaments'.

For serious lovemaking in the West today we normally get entirely naked, so ornamentation is something different and can be a lot of fun. There's the opportunity for the sort of flamboyance that would get you a lot of funny looks the rest of the time. The idea is both to create a sense of occasion and emphasize, rather than cover, the genitals, breasts and – for a man – muscles.

For *Kama Sutra*-style sex the following are essential for women:

- lots of bracelets on both wrists
- at least one bracelet on each upper arm
- bracelets around the ankles
- at least one necklace
- earrings
- some jewels, decorations or flowers in the hair which should be 'hanging loose'.

Here are some traditional and modern clothing ideas for women (who are otherwise naked, apart from jewellery). Wear:

- a short bolero
- a wide belt
- a choker and elbow-length gloves

- a suspender belt and a pair of boots
- a suspender belt with fishnet stockings and a half-cup bra
- a cowboy hat (and chaps, if you can get them).
- high heels.

The idea of ripping clothes off appeals to a lot of men and, as we'll see, a little boisterous physicality is entirely in keeping with the *Kama Sutra*, so don't throw your old clothes away – keep them for a session of some really ripping fun.

A man should wear the following jewellery:

- at least one bracelet on each wrist
- one bracelet on each ankle
- one bracelet on each upper arm
- a necklace.

A man should be naked apart from his jewellery and:

- headwear, such as a bandanna, scarf or hat
- a waistcoat (optional)
- a tie (optional).

As we'll see in Chapter 08, the ancient Indians did have a kind of 'jewellery' for the penis, whose main function was to provide additional stimulation. But there's no mention in the *Kama Sutra* of specifically erotic jewellery for women. Nowadays, however, there are nipple rings and shields as well as jewellery for the vulva, held in place by a tab inserted into the vagina just like a tampon. You can find these in some sex shops as well as on the internet.

Flowers

Both women and men also habitually wore garlands of flowers in Vatsyayana's time. For going out they would have worn whatever flowers in season had the best scent, perhaps jasmine, but for sex it was always yellow amaranth, because the flowers don't disintegrate as others do.

Have a go: make a garland

In the absence of yellow amaranth, carnations make an excellent garland. You'll need about four dozen for each one.

- Cut the stems off at the base of the flowers.
- Cut a length of thick cotton double the length of the garland, plus about 30cm.
- Thread the cotton onto a needle so the eye is in the middle.
- Take half the flowers. Pass the needle and thread through the centre of each one, going in at the bottom (calyx) and coming out at the top. Gently move the flowers along the thread.
- Take the remaining half. Pass the needle and thread through the centre of each one in the opposite direction, that's to say, down through the top of the flower and out through the calyx.
- Cut the needle off.
- You should now have all the flowers on the thread, half facing one way and half facing the other way, towards the first half.
- Tie the four ends.

You could also make a headband. You'll need some special materials, available in a craft shop or at a good florist.

- For the base of the headband, measure out a length of coiled floral wire sufficient to go around the head, plus 10cm.
- Twist a loop into one end of the wire.
- Bend the wire into shape.
- Wrap the wire with floral tape.
- Cut the stems at about 2.5cm from the flowers.
- Tape a short length of floral wire to each flower and stem to stiffen it and provide a means of attaching it to the headband.
- Tape the flowers to the headband.
- Adjust the headband on the person who'll be wearing it (if it's for yourself, you'll need someone to help you); pass the free end of the wire through the loop you made and bend it back to make a hook. If necessary, cut off any excess wire.

Henna and body paint

Quite often in Indian erotic art you'll see that the women have decorated their bodies with intricate patterns. And, indeed, colouring the body, as well as nails and teeth, was among the 64 arts. It was normally done only for very special occasions such as weddings but, for fun, you might like to try the same.

Traditionally, the designs were made with henna, known in India as *mehndi, mehandi, mylanchi* and various other names. In the West, henna has caught on as a long-lasting but temporary alternative to a tattoo. It creates its darkest effects where the skin is thickest, which is why you most often see it on hands and feet.

Henna is a shrub or small tree (*Lawsonia inermis*) whose leaves, when dried and powdered, become a powerful dye. You can buy it in craft shops, chemists, health shops and on the internet. Buy yours from a source with a rapid turnover because henna quickly goes stale, unless it's extremely well-packaged. When you get it home, store any henna you're not immediately using in an airtight container in the freezer. That way it will last for several years.

The quality of henna varies considerably as all natural products do. Although the plant is pruned back several times a year to produce a continuous crop, experts consider that the best comes from India, Pakistan and Yemen when harvested at the beginning of the monsoon season, as well as Morocco when harvested just after the first spring rains. A specialist supplier should be able to advise you.

Some suppliers try to 'improve' their henna artificially by adding green dye. To test yours, mix it with lemon juice and put it on a sheet of glass. If bright green dots appear after about 15 minutes then dye has been added.

Warning

Do not use so-called 'black henna', containing para-phenylenediamine, for body art. An extremely dangerous substance for the skin, it can cause permanent scarring and, in extreme cases, death.

No henna should be used on children under six.

Have a go

Your powder first needs to be sifted, mixed to a paste with lemon juice to release the dye, and then left to oxidize for anything from two hours to a day, depending on the temperature. The henna is applied using a plastic cone, a paint brush or a special container known as a jac bottle. Once the design is complete, the skin is wrapped in plastic for six to eight hours. A spray of water, lemon juice and sugar will aid penetration. The colour will deepen over two or three days and last from a week to a month.

But, unless you're an artist, how are you going to recreate those beautiful designs? In fact, it isn't as difficult as it seems because there is a way of 'cheating'. Don't buy stencils because they don't work. A better trick is to use old-fashioned carbon paper (make sure you buy the sort for pen/pencil use, not the kind used in typewriters). Here's what you do:

- Print out a design from the internet.
- Lay your design on top of the ink side of the carbon paper.
- Trace over the design with a hard pencil or biro using firm pressure.
- You will now have a copy of the design in carbon on the reverse side of your print-out.
- Cover the skin with deodorant from a glycerine-based deodorant stick.
- Press the carbon copy you've just made onto the skin; the carbon will come off, leaving a pattern onto which you can apply the henna.
- Henna the design.

Obviously, there's a whole art to the preparation and use of henna. If you're interested I'd recommend you to go on a course or at the very least, buy a book. For useful websites see 'Taking it further' at the end of this book. If you can't be bothered with henna, there are special body paints you can buy from art shops which last about three days. Alternatively, some tattoo parlours offer henna as an alternative to permanent tattoos.

A *Kama Sutra* body

Some of the positions of the *Kama Sutra* do call for a pretty supple body, and not just for the woman. Men commonly squatted to make love in ancient India, a position that Richard Burton likened to a 'bird' and said was 'impossible to Europeans'. In fact, it's far from impossible but it does become tiring fairly quickly. Yet all over the developing world, whenever a chair isn't available, men and women squat both for comfort and to save their clothes from the ground. It helps to have done it from childhood but, with practice, you can build up to quite a long time. For women it's the key, as we'll see later, to the position of Indrani. Give it a go next time you're out for a picnic.

Yoga is a good form of exercise for sex. Indeed, yoga *is* sex. The word is derived from the Sanskrit *Yuj* meaning to 'join' or 'unite'. In one form, it means joining with the Divine Spirit. In another sense, it could mean joining with another person.

Here are a few yoga-based exercises to prepare you for the sexual athletics ahead. The first is a variation on squatting.

- **Spread squats** – Stand with your feet slightly more than shoulder-width apart and, with your legs slightly bent, bend over and place yours hands on your feet. Now gradually straighten your legs as far as you can. This is your start position. From this position, with your head hanging, squat down then raise yourself once again into the start position, stretching your legs as far as you can. Exhale as you go down; inhale as you come up.

- **The Bow** – Lie on your stomach. Bend your knees and bring your feet as close to your buttocks as you can manage, so that you can reach behind and grab your ankles. Now begin to straighten your legs so that your body is pulled into an arch. This is your start position. Rock backwards, inhaling, then forwards, exhaling.

- **The Bridge** – Lie on your back with the soles of your feet on the floor, knees bent, and your arms stretched comfortably along the floor past your head, palms upwards. This is your start position. Now inhale as you lift your pelvis and back off the floor and hold for a few seconds. Exhale as you come back down.

- **Butterfly** – Sit on the floor with your thighs open, your knees bent and the soles of your feet pressed together and pulled back towards your groin. Put your hands on your feet. Your start position is sitting up, with your spine straight and your chest out. Now bend forward, exhaling, to drop your head as close to your toes as you can manage. Inhale as you return to the start position.

- **Half Lotus** – For this it helps to have generous buttocks and skinny legs. Anybody else – which is most of us – will have to struggle. Sit on the floor with your back straight and your legs out in front of you in a V-shape. Pull one foot back towards your groin and tuck it under the opposite thigh. Now bring the other foot back and manhandle it on top of the other thigh. If you should happen to be one of the rare rubber people who find it easy, try sitting with *both* feet on top of the thighs – that's the full lotus.

- *Supta Vajrasana* (**Kneeling Pose**) – It helps to be on something soft for this, so try it on your bed. At first it's also a good idea to have a partner to help you. Kneel with legs comfortably apart, sit on your feet and gradually ease yourself backwards, using your elbows for support, until your head and back are resting on the bed.

- **Sex Nerves** – Lie on your back, thighs apart, knees bent and the soles of your feet together. Inhale as you stroke your inner thighs from your knees up to your groin. Think of sucking up energy into your genitals. Exhale as you return your hands to your knees, but without touching yourself.

Couples exercises

Exercising together is a fun and intimate way of improving your co-ordination as a couple. Here are two exercises that you can make part of a bigger exercise routine or incorporate into your love play.

- **Standing Arches** – This is really exhilarating. Standing back to back, interlock your arms at the elbows. With knees bent, one of you now leans forward, stretching the other over his or her back. Unless you're both confident in your strength and suppleness, the toes of the partner being stretched should not leave the ground Hold the position and breathe deeply. Now do it the opposite way.

- **Leg Stretch** – Sit facing one another, legs wide open. The shorter of you places his or her feet against the other's ankles. Now grip each other's wrists. Take turns leaning back and pulling the other forward.

Weight

Some of the positions in the *Kama Sutra* are going to be pretty difficult if – man or woman – you're much heavier than you should be. Apart from which, being overweight means an increased risk of heart disease, high blood pressure and diabetes which, in turn, can lead to impaired sexual capacity.

Middle-aged men need to be particularly vigilant. Those so-called 'love handles' are more accurately 'anti-love handles'. That's because the fat cells around the waist cause excess production of something called aromatase enzyme, which converts testosterone to oestrogen. Testosterone is the 'male' sex hormone while oestrogen is the 'female' sex hormone. The result is anything from mild erectile dysfunction up to complete impotence.

There are two rules:

- Keep down the level of saturated fat in your meals – it immediately lowers testosterone for up to four hours.
- Keep your Body Mass Index (BMI) at 24 or lower.

Calculating your BMI is very simple. All you have to do is divide your weight in pounds by your height in inches and multiply by 10.

Example

You are 5' 10" tall which equals 70". You weigh 10 stones which equals 140 pounds. To find your BMI, begin by dividing 140 by 70. The answer is two. Now multiply by 10 and you see that your BMI is 20.

(To convert centimetres to inches divide by 2.54; to convert kilograms to pounds multiply by 2.2.)

This is not the place to go into nutrition in detail. If you are overweight you should consult your GP. The magic figure to remember is that 3,500 calories is equivalent to 1lb/450 grams of body weight. In order to lose 24lbs/11 kg in a year:

- eat 230 fewer calories a day (equivalent to an average pudding), or
- walk for 45 minutes a day, or
- have *Kama Sutra*-style sex for 45 minutes a day.

The PC muscle

The exquisite technique known as the 'pair of tongs' described in Chapter 11 is only possible if a woman has a well-developed PC muscle. It's also an important muscle for men. So, while we're on the subject of exercise we might as well strengthen the PC muscle, too.

In fact, it's not one muscle but a whole group of muscles with unpronounceable names like *ischiocavernosus*. So let's just stick with PC muscle. Okay?

The PC muscle runs from the pubic bone to the tailbone in women and men. It's what's holding your insides in place, especially, if you're a woman, your vagina. The stronger the muscle, the more powerful the orgasms you'll experience. On the other hand, weakness of the PC muscle leads, in extreme cases, to leakage of urine or incontinence. If you want to know how your PC muscle is doing, slip a finger into the entrance of your vagina and try squeezing it. Another test is to try interrupting the flow of urine. If you can't stop in mid-pee then the muscle is too weak.

The PC muscle also powers the male orgasm. If you're a man, you can try the same pee-test as a woman.

So, how do you strengthen this muscle? Both sexes can improve it simply by squeezing it several times a day. That's to say, contracting it exactly as you would when you feel the need to pee and there's nowhere to go. With clothes on it's completely invisible so you can do it any time, anywhere. In fact, you can do it while reading this, even if you're sitting on a train. Aim for three sessions a day, beginning with ten contractions each time and working up to 50 contractions.

The exercises will be far more powerful if there's a resistance to squeeze against. If you're a woman, an easy way of providing a resistance is to insert two lubricated fingers into your vagina, open them (as if making a V-sign) and then try to force them closed using your vagina (and, therefore, your PC muscle).

The *Kama Sutra* particularly mentions the women of the Andra country as having powerful PC muscles. Undoubtedly, they would have been using stone eggs, a practice that goes back thousands of years. Nowadays you can obtain them in jade as well as modern materials such as stainless steel. The idea is to pop a lubricated egg into the vagina and then use the vaginal muscles to move it up and down. Squeezing the perineum and vagina moves the egg up, while bearing down (as for a bowel movement) sends it down and out. Effective when properly done, the drawback with eggs is that since they provide no feedback it's easy to do the exercises ineffectively and, what's more, lose motivation.

Modern technology has provided a better if less aesthetically-pleasing option. These kinds of exercises are nowadays known as Kegel exercises after Dr Arnold Kegel who devised them as a non-surgical method of tackling urinary stress incontinence. Dr Kegel's method was particularly sophisticated because it involved an apparatus (the Kegel Perineometer), which provided a resistance, together with a dial to give the all-important biofeedback.

Dr Kegel's Perineometer went out of production years ago but there are modern equivalents. Look for a design that allows you to change the degree of resistance through a dozen or so settings using a series of springs. That way, you can increase the resistance as you get stronger and also monitor progress, which is good for morale.

Sources for these kinds of exercisers are given in 'Taking it further' at the end of this book.

Keeping motivated

Following the philosophy of the *Kama Sutra*, here are some suggestions to keep you motivated:

- Make exercise a ritual.
- Don't let the weather put you off – have alternatives for when it's too hot or too cold or too wet for your preferred sport.
- Exercise with friends, so you can encourage one another.
- Hang a scene from the *Kama Sutra* on the wall, showing the body you're aiming for.
- Enjoy your exercise – don't make it a chore.
- Play music while exercising at home.
- Set measurable and attainable goals and celebrate when you reach them.
- Keep an exercise diary.
- Make a list of all the exercise benefits you're hoping for and look at it regularly.

Summary

- The ancient Hindus had hygiene products like toothpaste and mouthwash.
- Both men and women used eyeliner and lipstick.
- Couples were seldom entirely naked for sex but always wore body jewellery and titillating clothing.
- You can make your own garlands of flowers to wear, just like the ancient Hindus.
- You can decorate your bodies with henna or body paint.
- Some simple exercises will get you fit for the Kama Sutra's more athletic positions.
- Women used to strengthen their PC muscles using stone 'eggs'.
- There are easy, modern ways to strengthen the PC muscle.

05

preparing the love chamber

In this chapter you will learn:
- how to furnish your bedroom
- how to create the right ambience
- what food and drink to serve.

This abode ... should be surrounded by a garden, and also contain two rooms, an outer and an inner one. The inner room should be occupied by the females, while the outer room, balmy with rich perfumes, should contain a bed, soft, agreeable to the sight, covered with a clean white cloth, low in the middle part, having garlands and bunches of flowers upon it, and a canopy above it, and two pillows, one at the top, another at the bottom ...

The *Kama Sutra*

In the *Kama Sutra* the furnishing of the 'pleasure room' is a matter of considerable importance. For most people it would have been the same as the bedroom (and even doubled as the lounge), but the wealthy had a completely separate room for sex. The older houses in Benares still have these 'love chambers', normally at the top of the property but sometimes as pavilions in the garden.

To read the *Kama Sutra*'s descriptions is to enter a world of sensuality, a culture in which sex has a central role. In Vatsyayana's time there were no televisions or computers and it was sex that was the main entertainment of the evening.

The *Kama Sutra* conjures up the erotically charged atmosphere with a few telling phrases: the room 'balmy with rich perfumes'; the bed 'agreeable to the sight' and draped with 'garlands and bunches of flowers'. Whenever you see illustrations of the *Kama Sutra*, whether modern or antique, there's always this emphasis on beautiful – sometimes four-poster – beds, colourful and elaborate cushions and intricate rugs as well as all the ancillaries such as flowers, decorations, ornaments, food and drink.

One thing the *Kama Sutra* doesn't mention about the bedroom is the temperature. Benares (modern-day Varanasi) is only just outside the tropics, but many of us live where the winters are pretty cool. Make sure your bedroom is at the sort of temperature you can comfortably be naked, say, around 21° C (70° F).

Furniture

Let's take a look at the room in more detail. According to the *Kama Sutra*, the main items of furniture should be:

• a bed, with a canopy over and pillows at each end
• a couch
• a round seat.

The bed

Just as today in the West, the bed seems to have been where most lovemaking would have taken place. The *Kama Sutra* says the bed should be soft, covered with a clean, white cloth and have a canopy over it.

Have a go: the *Kama Sutra* bed

Your bed is your most important piece of furniture. When you're choosing it don't just think of sleeping. Think of sex. There's a fashion for low beds but they're not very versatile when it comes to positions. The ideal is a bed with the top of the mattress at roughly knee height. That opens up all sorts of additional possibilities as we'll see later in the book. Nor is it a good idea to have anything that sticks out beyond the mattress – wooden surrounds, brass twiddles or whatever. A banged shin isn't a great prelude to lovemaking. It's also best to avoid anything sticking up at the foot of the bed. You may sometimes want to launch yourself from that end. Above all, make sure it's solid. Don't just lie on it in the shop, bounce up and down on it.

A canopy is essential for that romantic, Oriental ambience. As a minimum, all you need is a fixing point above the bed from which you can hang some material. This can then be tucked behind the bed head and around the sides a little way. If mosquitoes are a problem, mosquito netting that falls to the floor all around the bed will serve two purposes.

The couch

According to some commentators, it was actually on the 'couch' that the couple would have had sex, keeping the bed for sleeping. According to others, the couple would have made love in bed and then the man would have moved to the 'couch' to get some undisturbed sleep. In reality, it's unlikely there were rigid rules. Apart from that we don't really know what form the 'couch' would have taken.

Have a go: the *Kama Sutra* couch

If you have space in the bedroom you really want a couch that offers different possibilities from a bed. That means wide, comfortable and, above all, strong arms and back for lying over, face up or face down. The arms can also be used to support a woman's pelvis, *yoni* pointing at the ceiling. There's no question that, for sex, the traditional Chesterfield is a good design.

The round seat

The 'round seat' is something of a mystery. Some translators have referred to it as an additional bed, which seems unlikely. Another version has it as a round mat complete with extra cushions for support while playing dice ... or anything else. That seems quite possible. Or it may just have been a stool.

Have a go: the *Kama Sutra* round seat

The main thing is that this should be a prop that opens up yet further possibilities. A well-cushioned stool or pouffe is ideal. A round mat with plenty of cushions can do the same job. Nowadays there are even inflatable cushions specially designed to support you in a variety of sexual positions (see 'Taking it further' for suppliers).

Bits and pieces

The *Kama Sutra* gives a long list of the miscellaneous items serious lovers should have available in the bedroom:

- incense
- betel (and a box for spitting it out)
- unguent
- flowers, including those for scent and decoration, garlands of yellow amaranth flowers and necklaces of kurantaka flowers
- pots containing collyrium, fragrant substances and massage oils
- things used for perfuming the mouth, including lemon bark
- a vina (lute) encrusted with ivory
- a board for drawing
- a board for playing with dice.

Nearby there should be talking birds in cages; and in the garden a whirling swing and a common swing.

Incense

Incense has been used for several thousand years and the joss stick, far from being a convenient invention for the 1960s, has existed for at least 2,000 years. Incense is specifically mentioned in the Vedas. It's easy to imagine how it all started: seated round their camp fires, people would have noticed that certain types of wood burned with a more fragrant smoke than others.

Incense was believed to have magical properties. When it comes to sex there's no doubt that certain aromas are a 'turn-off' while others – the dark, mysterious ones – are a 'turn-on'.

Have a go: make your own incense

You can buy incense very easily nowadays in the form of cones and joss sticks. But it's worth making your own because:

- a personalized incense is something very special
- you can ensure it's an aroma that turns you both on.

Health shops and herbalists should have what you need, especially those specializing in Ayurvedic medicine; if not, take a look on the internet (see 'Taking it further'). Above all, you need something to keep your aromatics burning slowly and steadily. Traditionally, that was the role of 'makko', which was made from the bark of the *Machillus thunbergii* tree. If you can't get hold of any makko try saltpetre (potassium nitrate) which is used in commercial incense products.

As for the aroma, try anything that appeals to you. Sandalwood is one of the best and easiest because it burns with very little makko. Easily available ingredients include clove, cinnamon and spikenard (an aromatic Indian plant).

If you can't find your ingredients in powder form you'll have to grind them yourself. Use a hand-cranked coffee mill rather than an electric one because it preserves the aromas better. Sieve the various powders together, including the makko, add some warm water and knead into a dough. Forming it into cones is easiest but you could also try rolling the dough out and cutting it into thin strips. Leave your incense to dry very slowly. Don't be impatient. It will take at least a week.

Be generous with your incense but don't overdo it. A cone in a safe place either side of the bed and another elsewhere in the room is about right.

Betel

Recommended throughout the *Kama Sutra* before (and after) sex, betel is a mixture of leaves and nuts which, rather curiously, come from two different plants. According to mythology, a strange creeper was found growing in an urn in which Amrut or ambrosia had been stored. The god Vishnu ordered

Dhanvantari to examine it and the distinctive taste of betel leaves (a mixture of peppery and minty) was thus discovered.

In reality the betel creeper doesn't grow on ambrosia but on the areca tree (*Areca Catechu*), which resembles the coconut palm and produces huge clusters of hazel-sized nuts. It was perhaps inevitable that someone would find out what happened when the nuts and the leaves were eaten together. The answer is: quite a lot. Westerners who try it for the first time report a powerful effect. They feel more alert and more vigorous to the point of euphoria, hot, sweaty and sexually aroused. For maximum effect lime powder can be added (from cooking coral over a bonfire for several days), together with various aromatics to improve the flavour (such as cardamom, camphor, tobacco or nutmeg). The wealthy used ground pearls in place of coral, together with whipped butter and saffron.

Have a go

Betel is still widely chewed all over India and South-East Asia today, but it's addictive, causes withdrawal symptoms and, what's more, habitual use stains the teeth red and eventually black, which is hardly very alluring.

Instead, you might like to share a glass of champagne, which is the Western equivalent for a romantic occasion. Indian erotic paintings frequently show one of the lovers holding a glass or even being passed something to drink by a servant. The ancient Indians certainly had wine as well as a kind of mead and some sort of rum flavoured with cardamom, aloes and cinnamon. If you don't like champagne or any other alcohol, some traditional Indian drinks are given below. Whatever you drink, make sure you serve it with the same ceremony that betel was once served. It's all part of the fun and sense of occasion. Open the bottle with all the proper paraphernalia and pour some into an elegant long-stemmed glass. Some lovers like to take a mouthful then 'kiss' it into the mouths of their partners.

Some traditional Indian drinks

Thandai

Ingredients:
16 fl oz/50cl of cold skimmed milk or soya
1 pod of cardamom seeds finely ground
12 blanched almonds soaked overnight
1 tbs sugar

Combine all the ingredients in an electric blender and serve well chilled.

Sweet lassi
Ingredients:
4 fl oz/125ml of plain yoghurt
12 fl oz/375ml of ice-cold water
1 tbs sugar

Combine all the ingredients in an electric blender (three seconds) and serve well chilled. As an alternative, you can serve salty lassi by replacing the sugar with salt, according to taste.

Lime flavoured with ginger
Ingredients:
10 tbs freshly squeezed lime juice
8 tbs sugar
1 tsp finely grated fresh ginger
Water to taste
Ice cubes

Stir the lime juice, sugar and ginger together in a bowl until the flavour is right. Pour into glasses through a strainer (to remove the ginger) and add the water and ice cubes.

Music

The *Kama Sutra* says there should be a vina or lute 'hanging from a peg'. Obviously, in Vatsyayana's time there weren't any radios or CDs so, if you wanted music while making love, you had to provide it yourself. Not easy. But an Indian erotic painting dating from around the time the Arbuthnot/Burton edition of the *Kama Sutra* was published shows how it was done.

The man is reclining with his head resting on a large red cushion while his lover sits astride him, his *lingam* in her *yoni*, while she also plays to him. It's a nice idea and if you have any musical skills at all you should definitely try it.

Have a go: music while making love

It helps to play something small like a flute or ukulele but even sex at the piano is definitely feasible. The least practical instrument is the cello. Think about it!

Most of us will have to leave it to the professionals. Without any doubt, music enhances sex and helps prolong the mood afterwards. Basically, it acts on the same parts of the brain that sex itself does. Whether or not Indian music turns you on is partly a question of familiarity. To Western ears it seems to lack direction. That's a reflection of the Hindu philosophy that things don't have a beginning and an end but are cyclical and eternal. And that's a great advantage in the bedroom, otherwise lovemaking is punctuated by the progression from one track to the next. If you're not used to it, start off with a fusion of Western and Indian styles. See 'Taking it further' for suggestions.

Paintings

Vatsyayana doesn't mention erotic paintings in the bedroom but by the time of the *Ananga Ranga*, about 1,000 years later, they were an integral part of the décor of any 'love chamber'. If you ever have the chance to visit some of the great old houses in Varanasi and to enter the 'pleasure room' you'll see erotic frescoes on the walls.

Not many people could afford that today but original Indian erotic watercolours can be bought relatively inexpensively on the internet.

Have a go: your own erotic pictures

In these days of digital cameras and home computers it's very easy to make your own erotic pictures. You can photograph one another and, with the aid of the time-delay feature, also photograph yourselves making love. It would be fun to do it in the Indian style with all the paraphernalia. You'll probably have to have quite a few attempts before you get any usable pictures but in the digital age that doesn't really matter.

It can be a good idea to mount your personal erotic photographs in double-sided frames, with something innocuous on the other side. It avoids awkwardness if, for example, children should go into the bedroom, but it also stops them losing their power to arouse. Only turn them round when you intend to make love.

Mirrors

Yashodhara's commentary to the *Kama Sutra* says there should be a mirror at the head of the bed and other commentators say there should also be mirrors on the surrounding walls. It's an exciting idea. To be able to see yourselves making love is highly arousing.

Have a go

For some 'quick kama' you could just bring a mirror close to the bed and lean it somewhere useful. But the ideal is a mirror permanently fixed to the wall behind the bed and angled slightly downwards. If you don't want it to be obvious to anyone else what the mirror is actually for, you could hinge the frame along the bottom edge and keep the mirror flush against the wall when it's not in use. When you want to see yourselves making love you can angle it by means of a cord attached to the wall and running through an eye on the top edge of the frame.

Of course, technology has provided more modern ways of going about things. If anything, a camcorder linked to a television is even more exciting, partly for the satisfaction of curiosity and partly for the *frisson* of being 'watched', even if it is only by a machine. You don't have to record anything if you don't want to, you can simply use the television as a monitor.

Alternatively, you might like to have the recording playing the next time you're making love. Some men like to use one as a backdrop to masturbation, known in ancient India as *simhakranta* or 'seizing the lion'.

Erotic films

Erotic films obviously didn't exist when the *Kama Sutra* was written but, if they had, Vatsyayana would undoubtedly have been recommending them.

People often say that sex films are 'boring'. Well, it all depends on the film and the mood you're in when you view them. It's a little bit like laughter. If you're not willing to laugh, the funniest comedian in the world will leave you unmoved. But when you feel in the mood to laugh the most trivial joke can have you rolling about on the floor.

It's exactly the same with a sex film. The director doesn't expect you to watch it from start to finish. He expects you to be rolling about on the floor, either on your own or with your partner. Those interminable scenes are there for you to masturbate to or make love to. If they only lasted a few seconds you wouldn't have time for either.

It's a fact that every normal person is excited by seeing images of other people having sex, whether they admit it or not. But it's equally true that different people react very differently to the same scene.

Some people like to see lovemaking from a little distance. Others like the camera to be right up close. So it can be difficult to find erotic films that will appeal equally to two people. You probably won't find anything suitable among the hardcore titles in your sex shop. Look instead in your local rental outlet or search for 'couples friendly films' on the internet (see 'Taking it further' for addresses).

Food and aphrodisiacs

Sex, *Kama Sutra* style, could go on a long time, which is why Vatsyayana says food as well as drink should be available in the bedroom. And, of course, it helped all the more if the food had aphrodisiac qualities.

The science of aphrodisiacs was known as *vrishhya yoga*. In Vatsyayana's time, all kinds of plants and magic spells were said to make women fall in or out of love, increase desire, turn women into sex slaves and increase sexual vigour. Many of them are complete rubbish, such as throwing 'the excrement of a monkey upon a maiden' to stop her being given in marriage to anybody else. Although, come to think of it, she might not be very popular afterwards.

Did any of them work? Well, if you're comparing with a modern drug such as Viagra then the effect would have been very disappointing. But some of the substances and recipes do seem to have a mild short-term effect. Interestingly, there are others that have a significant long-term effect. In other words, they were a tonic, the sort of food supplement we'd nowadays get from the health shop. Given that the medicinal effects of food are only now being recognized in the West, this was a significant insight from the ancient Indians.

In any event, you have to eat something and foods that are reputed to have aphrodisiac qualities are fun.

Unfortunately, many of the plants mentioned by Vatsyayana can't now be identified with any certainty. It doesn't help that in Sanskrit many plants had several different names. Uchchata, for example, is sometimes translated as garlic, sometimes as kidney beans and sometimes as other things. Personally, I'd go along with garlic because the active ingredient, allicin, lowers 'bad' LDL cholesterol, which can lead to atherosclerosis in the pudendal and penile arteries. So it's true to say that garlic is a kind of aphrodisiac because it can keep the blood flowing to the penis (and, come to that, the clitoris). What's more, men who aren't used to raw garlic often report an effect within an hour or so of eating a couple of cloves.

Similarly, three different plants are nowadays called guduchi, but Vatsyayana almost certainly meant *Tinospora cordifolia* rather than either *Menispermum cordifolium* or *Cissampelos pareira* and it's an ingredient in 'men's health' tablets today.

One of the most interesting plants mentioned by Vatsyayana is a member of the asparagus family, *Asparagus racemosus*, a shrub up to three metres high, which grows on the plains and foothills of India. Modern science has identified a huge variety of chemicals and, yes, it's still prescribed today as an aphrodisiac as well as for a whole range of conditions. So that's another success for Vatsyayana.

Other recipes include milk, sugar, ghee (clarified butter), honey and *kshirikapoli*, which some translators say was a type of onion. That makes sense. Similar recipes were also used in the Middle East and frequently appeared in the *Arabian Nights*, which Burton, as its translator, would have known very well.

Onions certainly have the magical ability to boost 'good' HDL cholesterol in the blood while depressing 'bad' LDL cholesterol. Over time that would certainly protect the circulation and, therefore, the ability of erectile tissue to erect. What's more, the sugar in the recipes would have facilitated the release of serotonin, which helps combat anxiety, a common cause of poor sexual performance. Serotonin can also reduce the urge to ejaculate so that a man might, as the *Kama Sutra* puts it, 'be able to enjoy innumerable women'.

Have a go: make your own aphrodisinacks

Like everything else, your aphrodisinacks (aphrodisiac snacks) should be beautifully presented. It can be great fun to pop them into one another's mouths, even more fun to pass them from mouth to mouth, and the greatest fun of all to do it actually while having sex. But never give someone an aphrodisiac without their knowledge.

Chillies

Chillies were introduced by the Portuguese and aren't native to India, but they've become an essential part of the Indian kitchen. Part of the fun is that you never know how hot a pepper is going to be until you taste it. Cook them lightly in oil and serve them on a plate sprinkled with a little salt.

Folklore all over the world has chilli peppers as aphrodisiacs, probably because the pain on the tongue causes the release of endorphins, just as sex does. So one thing reinforces the other.

A word of warning: chilli 'essence' will do the same to a *lingam* or *yoni* as it does to a tongue, so be careful with fingers and oral sex afterwards.

Milk with garlic

The *Kama Sutra* says that: 'A man obtains sexual vigour by drinking milk mixed with sugar, the root of the uchchata plant, the pipar chaba and liquorice.'

Uchchata, as we've already seen, was probably garlic and *pipar chaba* was white pepper. So warm some milk in a pan together with a stick or two of liquorice. Crush two garlic cloves into the milk together with sugar to taste. Remove from the heat and season with white pepper.

Milk with onions

Another Kama Sutra recipe recommends a drink made of milk, *kshirikapoli* and *svayamgupta* roots. *Kshirikapoli*, as already mentioned, is believed to have been a kind of onion. *Svayamgupta* appears to have been the plant known to us today as *Mucuna pruriens*, which, like *Tribulus terrestris*, is still in use as an aphrodisiac.

Ingredients:
1 large glass of milk
1 large onion
1 *Mucuna pruriens* tablet (available on the internet)
Sugar

Pound the onion to extract the juice, crush the tablet. Add the juice and the crushed tablet to the milk and warm in a saucepan. The more sugar you add, the calmer you're likely to feel and, if you're a man, the less urgently you'll want to ejaculate.

Barley for bonking

The *Kama Sutra* says that sexual stamina will be increased 'if the powder of the seed of the *shvadaushtra* plant and the flour of barley are mixed together in equal parts and ... eaten every morning'.

Barley may not seem very exciting but, in the long term, it's almost magical. Compounds in barley actually stifle the liver's production of the 'bad' LDL cholesterol that damages blood vessels. Since most of the cholesterol in the body is actually produced by the body, eating barley is a far more powerful weapon for improving circulation than simply cutting down on high-cholesterol foods. So barley is a long-term tonic for getting blood to the genitals, and it's intriguing that the ancient Indians already knew this.

The *shvadaushtra* plant, on the other hand, works in a completely different, almost immediate, way. It seems to have been the plant *Tribulus terrestris*, which is still used as an aphrodisiac today. Vatsyayana's recipe is rather boring so here's a more tasty version.

Ingredients:
Handful of barley grits
1 clove garlic
1 *Tribulus terrestris* tablet (available on the internet)
Some diced cucumber
Half a cup of yoghurt
Fresh mint leaves
Olive oil
Lemon
Salt and pepper

Soak the barley grits for an hour, squeeze dry and spread on a plate. Sprinkle with olive oil, a squeeze of lemon and salt and pepper to taste. Crush the Tribulus terrestris tablet and the garlic over the barley. Add the cucumber. Top off with yoghurt and decorate with the fresh mint leaves.

Oysters

Oysters have long been considered the ultimate snack for a night of love. So even though they're not mentioned by the *Kama Sutra* they can't be ignored. The truth is that oysters contain enormous quantities of zinc, and zinc is an important constituent of semen. In fact, about half the recommended daily allowance (RDA) for men is lost with every ejaculation, and not many men even consume the RDA. Men with inadequate zinc don't produce enough testosterone and can even become impotent, so it's with good reason that many Oriental sex gurus have warned against too frequent ejaculation.

There's another point. Zinc concentration in a normal prostate gland is three to ten times higher than in other tissues. In the cancerous prostate, on the other hand, zinc levels are very low. It seems that malignant prostate cells are unable to accumulate it, but there's evidence that a high zinc intake, as it were, forces the malignant cells to take up zinc and, in so doing, to increase apoptosis, which is the process of programmed cell death.

So zinc is vital, and the biggest natural source of zinc is a plate of oysters. About three ounces will give you 63mg of the stuff. No other food comes near, so for anyone with a deficiency, oysters could, indeed, be said to be an aphrodisiac.

Have a go

Make sure your oysters are alive. That's absolutely essential. A dead oyster will give you food poisoning. If the shell opens easily the oyster is dead; if you have to struggle it's alive. So how do you open a live oyster? Get yourself a proper oyster knife and, holding the oyster on a table with the flatter shelf uppermost, insert the tip of the blade into the small hole in the hinge. Twist the blade sharply (some people wear a glove on their other hand in case the knife slips). Discard the upper shell and pass the knife under the oyster (which will kill it). Arrange your oysters on a bed of crushed ice, without spilling the liquid in the lower shell. Serve with quarters of lemon, freshly ground black pepper or tabasco sauce.

If you don't like oysters, then the easiest way to get a zinc boost is to take a zinc supplement. Around 15mg of zinc a day would be right for most people and you'll need to balance it with 1mg of copper.

Mung dal

Finally, here's a very popular Indian snack for which no aphrodisiac qualities are claimed. It is, however, easy to prepare in advance.

Ingredients:
7oz/200 g mung dal
Salt
Fresh black pepper

Wash the mung dal (split mung beans) in several changes of water and leave to soak for six to eight hours. Dry. Heat some oil in a deep pan and lower two handfuls of the dal into the oil in a sieve until golden. Empty onto kitchen paper. Continue until all the dal are cooked. Season with salt and pepper and store until needed.

Summary

- Every detail of your bedroom should be worked out for sex.
- Put some sort of canopy up over the bed for that Oriental feeling.
- The bedroom furniture should also include a couch and a comfortable, low stool or pouffe.
- Always light incense for making love.
- Always serve drinks.
- Always put on some suitable music.
- Hang some erotic pictures on the walls – they could include you.
- A mirror by the bed can be extremely exciting.
- Serve aphrodisiac snacks.

06

foreplay and oral sex

In this chapter you will learn:
- the ancient Indian style of foreplay
- how to perform oral sex
- how to perform 'the congress of a crow'.

Some women of the harem, when they are amorous, do the acts of the mouth on the yonis of one another, and some men do the same thing with women. The way of doing this (kissing the yoni) should be known from kissing the mouth.

The *Kama Sutra*

Nowadays we don't divide sex up into 'foreplay' and 'intercourse' in the way we did even just a few years back. For some of us, occasionally or even routinely, oral sex *is* our style of sex. But in Vatsyayana's time, foreplay was always a prelude to penetration. There's no mention of women having orgasms during 'foreplay'. A couple compensated for that by lengthy intercourse in a variety of positions, as we'll see in Chapters 09 and 10. But, for now, we're going to concentrate on foreplay.

If use of fingers, lips and tongues was less intense than it often is nowadays, love games and different styles of kissing and cuddling were far more inventive.

According to the *Kama Sutra*, a woman will know she's turned her partner on if he looks at her in such a way as to cause the state of his mind to be known to her; he should pull about his moustache, make a sound with his nails, cause his own ornaments to tinkle, bite his lower lip, and make various other signs of that description.

The man will know his opening moves are going well by the following signs: her body relaxes, she closes her eyes, she puts aside all bashfulness and shows increased willingness to unite the two organs as closely together as possible.

Vatsyayana says that whatever is done by one of the lovers should be returned. It's a good piece of advice for overcoming any embarrassment about asking for what you want. Agree with your partner that you'll follow Vatsyayana's rule and then if you wish to have your nipples played with, you first play with your partner's nipples, and so on.

Chat up *Kama Sutra* style

The *Kama Sutra* quotes the sage Ghotakamukha as advising that 'though a man loves a girl ever so much, he never succeeds in winning her without a great deal of talking'.

So what should a man or, come to that, a woman, actually say?

- Say how attractive your partner is.
- Say how much you love him or her.
- Say how excited you feel.
- Describe what you're going to do.
- Describe the things you want your partner to do.

If you whisper all these things into your partner's ear it will work all the better.

The embraces

The *Kama Sutra* is very particular about the way a couple should embrace. First of all there should be just a slight and tantalizing touching of bodies. Then the woman should 'pierce' the man with her breasts. He responds by taking hold of them. Vatsyayana stresses the importance of a man being able to undo the 'knot' of a woman's 'undergarments' with one hand. The modern equivalent would be being able to undo a bra strap with one hand. If you can't do it, get practising.

Next you rub up against one another. It's even more sexy if one of you is pushed back against a wall.

The *Kama Sutra* describes two very special embraces, both done by women:

- *Jataveshtitaka* is translated as 'the twining of a creeper'. The woman literally wraps herself around the man and pulls his head down for a kiss.
- *Vriskshadhirudhaka* is translated as 'climbing a tree'. The woman puts one foot on her partner's foot and the other on his thigh and with the help of an arm around his neck 'climbs up' for a kiss.

Embraces in bed

It has to be remembered that, in many houses, the bed would have doubled as a couch, so the fact that a woman was sitting on the bed didn't necessarily mean she wanted sex. Hence Vatsyayana's advice: 'While the woman is lying on his bed, and is as it were abstracted by his conversation, he should loosen the knot of her undergarments, and when she begins to dispute with him he should overwhelm her with kisses. Then when his *lingam* is erect he should touch her with his hands in various places, and gently manipulate various parts of the body.'

If the woman still wasn't 'in the mood', then the man should 'place his hands between her thighs' and 'get his hands upon her breasts'.

This smacks of seduction or even worse. But it has to be remembered that, to some extent, it was, on both sides, a game. In fact, it's a game that nowadays can just as easily be reversed. There's no reason a woman shouldn't equally seduce a man by, say, putting a hand in one of his trouser pockets or sliding a hand inside his trousers.

In bed there were, once again, several special ways of embracing:

- *Tila-Tandulaka*
- *Kshiraniraka*
- the embrace of the forehead
- the embrace of the breasts
- the embrace of the *jaghana*.

Tila-Tandulaka translates as 'the mixture of sesame seed with rice'. The Arbuthnot/Burton edition of the *Kama Sutra* says you encircle the arms and thighs of your partner with your own arms and thighs. The Doniger/Kakar translation, on the other hand, describes it as 'wrestling', which sounds like a lot more fun.

Kshiraniraka translates as 'milk and water'. The image is of the two liquids mingling with one another until they're indistinguishable, and this is the same thing with flesh. You and your partner squeeze yourselves together, 'as if ... entering into each other's bodies' without thinking of 'any pain or hurt'.

The embrace of the forehead simply involves, well, nothing more exciting than pressing your foreheads together. But it's cosy. Noses, mouths and chins tend to follow. For the 'embrace of the breasts' the woman presses her breasts as hard as she can against the man's chest.

In the embrace of the *jaghana,* Arbuthnot and Burton say the man gets on top of the woman, while Doniger and Kakar say the woman gets on top of the man. Either will do very nicely. *Jaghana* is one of those words that can be translated in various ways. Arbuthnot and Burton sometimes translate it as 'middle parts', while Daniélou translates it more specifically as 'ass' or even 'vagina'. The essential is that pubic areas are ground against one another, while hands dig into buttocks. While you're doing it you can also kiss (of which more below) as well as scratch, bite and slap (of which more in the next chapter).

Kissing

The *Kama Sutra* dedicates an entire chapter to kissing, with at least half a dozen styles for mouth-to-mouth kissing alone:

- the nominal kiss – little more than a brushing of lips
- the throbbing kiss – now the lips get active
- the touching kiss – now the tongues get active
- the clasping kiss – you take both of your partner's lips between your own
- the greatly pressed kiss – you squeeze your partner's lips into a little ball using the circle made by your own thumb and forefinger, then you kiss
- the fighting of the tongue – you use your tongue vigorously inside your partner's mouth.

In addition, Vatsyayana suggests kissing the forehead, hair, cheeks, eyes, chest, breasts, the joints of the thighs, the armpits and, with certain reservations, the vulva and the penis.

And as ever, he likes to make a game of things: 'As regards kissing, a wager may be laid as to which will get hold of the lips of the other first. If the woman loses, she should pretend to cry, should keep her lover off by shaking her hands, and turn away from him and dispute with him, saying, "Let another wager be laid." If she loses this a second time, she should appear doubly distressed, and when her lover is off his guard or asleep, she should get hold of his lower lip, and hold it in her teeth, so that it should not slip away; and then she should laugh, make a loud noise, deride him, dance about and say whatever she likes in a joking way.'

As to the wager itself Vatsyayana made no suggestions, so here are some ideas to get you going. The loser has to:

- masturbate while the other watches
- lick his/her partner all over
- make love to his/her partner, who just lays back and enjoys it.

Have a go: foreplay and lubrication

The *Kama Sutra* mentions the application of 'unguent' or, as we'd say nowadays, lubrication. Copious lubrication is the secret of great sex and the *yoni* and the *lingam* produce their own up to a point. Maximizing it is one of the skills and aims of foreplay. But there are times something extra is needed:

- when stimulating the *yoni* or *lingam* with fingers
- when using a sex toy
- sometimes at the beginning of intercourse
- during lengthy intercourse
- for older couples
- for *adhorata* (anal stimulation and penetration)

Saliva is readily available and about the right viscosity. Some people object on the grounds that saliva carries bacteria, but taken in the context of everything that goes on during sex that hardly seems logical. Light salad oils from the kitchen (such as grape seed) will do at a pinch, but remember that oil should never be used with latex condoms as it can make holes in them; apart from that, oil could encourage infections in the vagina.

The best option, especially for sex toys and older couples, is a commercial sex lubricant. There are masses to choose from (in a sex shop or on the internet). Try them out and see which one you enjoy the best. Lubricants containing silicone are extremely long lasting but some people say they just don't feel 'wet'. Oil-based lubricants, as already mentioned, can damage latex condoms. Good water-based lubricants have the most natural feel but you'll have to keep replenishing them as they dry out quickly.

If you've never used lubricants before you'll almost certainly find they enhance your sexual pleasure.

Tip: apply lubricant *after* oral sex, unless you're certain you like the taste.

Oral sex

Oral sex was known as *auparishtaka* and translated by Burton and Arbuthnot as 'mouth congress'. It's clear that even in the hedonistic world of the ancient Hindus *auparishtaka* was frowned upon by some. Vatsyayana, for his part, believed that in sexual matters everybody should act according to 'his own inclination'.

Fellatio

According to Vatsyayana, fellatio was something that was only done by 'unchaste and wanton women'. As for men, 'mouth congress' was something that 'should never be done by a learned Brahman, by a minister that carries on the business of a state, or by a man of good reputation'. So it wasn't much fun being any of those.

Nowadays in the West, it's considered a normal part of sex play, whether you're a 'wanton' woman or a minister or not. So that's one way we're less hung up than the ancient Indians. Vatsyayana also debated whether or not *auparishtaka* was 'clean' in the religious sense. He concluded that 'the mouth of a woman is clean for kissing and suchlike things at the time of sexual intercourse'. Apparently it wasn't 'clean' at other times.

But Vatsyayana has a sly afterthought: 'these things being done secretly, and the mind of the man being fickle, how can it be known what any person will do at any particular time and for any particular purpose?'

Those who fancied it, but whose partners weren't sufficiently 'wanton', could call for 'shampooers' – eunuchs who would provide a massage and quite a lot more.

Have a go: *auparishtaka* on men

There were eight different techniques:

- The nominal congress: gently take hold of the base of your partner's *lingam* in your fist, slip your lips over the glans and move your head around.
- Biting the sides: gently take hold of the glans with the fingers and thumb of one hand, then run your lips along the shaft giving gentle bites.
- Pressing outside: take the glans between your lips, squeeze with pursed lips and withdraw.
- Pressing inside: take the glans right inside your mouth, purse your lips and withdraw.
- Kissing: take hold of your partner's *lingam* and kiss it as if kissing the lower lip.
- Rubbing: run your tongue all over the *lingam*, including the shaft, frenulum, glans and the urethral outlet.
- Sucking a mango fruit: take half the length of the *lingam* into your mouth and kiss and suck vigorously.
- Swallowing up: take the whole *lingam* into your mouth as if you were actually going to swallow it.

Cunnilingus

Vatsyayana writes that for the sake of great oral sex, 'courtesans abandon men possessed of good qualities, liberal and clever, and become attached to low persons, such as slaves and elephant drivers'. The technique, he says, is the same as for 'kissing the mouth'. He also points out that the people of the Lat country kiss the joints of the thighs. That's a good place to start.

Have a go: *auparishtaka* on women

Begin, like the people of the Lat country, by working your way along the creases of the thighs. Then kiss and lick the whole vulva.

Once your partner is aroused, turn your head sideways and follow Vatsyayana's instructions for kissing, treating the smooth inner lips of the *yoni* just as the lips of the mouth, and treating the vagina just as the interior of the mouth.

- The greatly pressed *yoni* kiss: using your fingers, gently squeeze your partner's labia together into a little mound and kiss and suck them.
- The throbbing *yoni* kiss: take each of the inner lips in turn and caress between your own lips.
- The touching *yoni* kiss: use your tongue on the inner lips and follow with long sweeping strokes from one end of the vulva to the other.
- The *yoni* tongue fight: push your tongue inside your partner's vagina as far as you can manage.

Vatsyayana and the clitoris

Vatsyayana didn't specifically mention the clitoris so it may well be that he hadn't discovered it. Nowadays, most people know that the clitoris is the little knob above the entrance to the vagina, where the inner lips meet. But there's still quite a bit of confusion between the clitoris itself (also known as the glans), the hood that covers the clitoris, and the shaft that leads to the hood.

At the beginning of foreplay you can kiss and lick the whole thing and gently suck it between your lips. But then you'll need to be more precise. The clitoris is actually the tiny little 'ball' under and normally concealed by the hood, which is why quite a lot of people think the hood is the clitoris. In most women the clitoris is only about the size of a lentil when excited so it's not surprising if it gets missed.

In fact, even the hood is extremely sensitive so if that's what you've been rubbing your partner will have been having a very good time. But the clitoris is *even more* sensitive than that.

Unless your partner has a larger than average clitoris, you'll have to manually retract the hood to get at it. The easiest way at first is to use the forefinger of one hand (nail well trimmed) to gently push the hood back. If you've done it correctly, you'll now see the tiny organ standing out a brighter pink than the rest. Use the tip of your tongue or the forefinger of your other hand for stimulation. (When you get good at it you'll be able to both hold the hood and stimulate with the same hand, leaving the other free for more fun.)

Remember that the clitoris is extremely sensitive. Too much pressure can hurt rather than excite. Gentle but rapid stimulation using only the tiniest of movements is enough to give many women a powerful orgasm. Just 'vibrate' your fingertip. Indeed, after an orgasm, many women say the clitoris is too delicate to be touched any more.

The elephant's trunk

Vatsyayana says: 'The man should rub the *yoni* of the woman with his hand and fingers (as the elephant rubs anything with his trunk) before engaging in congress, until it is softened, and after that is done he should proceed to put his *lingam* into her.'

Exactly what elephants have to do with it wouldn't be clear without Yashodhara's commentary, which explains that the three middle fingers are bunched together for insertion into the *yoni*. Like this, with the middle finger protruding slightly, they resemble the tip of the elephant's trunk.

Before doing anything, your fingernails should be closely trimmed. Begin by inserting just one *lubricated* finger into your partner's vagina. Gently explore inside. The rough area on the front wall of the vagina, just inside the opening, is the G-spot, of which more in Chapter 11. The little rubbery protrusion at the far end is the cervix, that's to say the opening into the uterus or womb. Some women quite enjoy having it caressed. Either side of the cervix are little hollows, beyond which lie the ovaries. When your partner says 'ouch' during intercourse it's because your penis has hit the end of one of these hollows and bumped an ovary.

As you're exploring, ask your partner if there are any areas which feel particularly good. Now you can progress to two fingers. They're less useful for exploring but moving them gently in and out creates a nice sensation. Only when the entrance to the vagina is fully relaxed should you insert the 'elephant's trunk', well smothered in lubricant. Be sensitive. Three fingers together are quite large and the knuckles can stick out at awkward angles. Done gently and well it can be very arousing. Done badly it's uncomfortable and even painful.

Oral sex positions

Most people associate 'positions' with intercourse and tend to approach oral sex in a more casual way. But skilful lovers know that specific postures can considerably enhance the pleasures of *auparishtaka*. Without the need to bring two sets of genitals together, oral sex allows for considerable freedom. The best positions for receiving oral sex are the ones that create the maximum muscular tension.

The *Kama Sutra* describes what it calls the 'congress of a crow'. Yashodhara says the name comes from the way you 'peck' at one-another's genitals. Another theory is that the word for 'crow' has the same root as a word meaning 'excess of passion'. We call it '69'.

The congress of a crow

The idea is to lie so you can simultaneously lick and suck one another's genitals. That is, the man and woman lie so that they can each stimulate the other's genitals with their mouths. There are three basic positions for 69. You can both lie on your sides, with your heads resting on your partner's inner thighs. The man can lie on his back and the woman can be on top. Or the woman can lie on her back and the man can get on top. It's a wonderful way of giving simultaneous stimulation. The only drawback is that the woman's tongue is on the 'wrong' side of the penis. That's to say, she can't use her tongue against the frenulum and underside of the glans which is the most sensitive part.

Vatsyayana makes no other suggestions for positions for oral sex so here are some, in the spirit of the *Kama Sutra*.

The standing crow

This is a position inspired by the marvellous erotic sculptures at Khajuraho, India, dating from around the 11th century CE. Essentially, it's the same as the congress of a crow except that the man is standing up and the woman is suspended upside-down. So it requires quite a lot of strength and agility. The easiest way to get into position is for the woman to kneel on the edge of the bed with her head and hands resting on it. The man then stands on the floor behind her, lifts her legs, rests her thighs over his shoulders and puts his arms around her. Her *yoni* should be right in front of his mouth. He now moves gently away from the bed and his partner helps support herself by putting her arms around him. She should be able to take his *lingam* into her mouth. If she needs extra support he can put a hand under her shoulder.

Why would anybody want to do it? Well, it's something you can do without needing anywhere comfortable to lie down. Blood rushing to the woman's head can enhance sensation. And it's just fun, which is what the *Kama Sutra* is all about.

The widely opened position

This is one of the positions for which the *Kama Sutra* recommended having a low stool in the bedroom (see Chapter 05) and we'll be meeting it again when we get onto intercourse. For receiving oral sex either the man or the woman can try it. Simply sit on the stool and lie back so that your feet and your head (supported by a pillow) are on the floor on opposite sides. Your partner kneels between your thighs.

If you prefer the bed, the easiest way of getting into the position is simply to lie face up and then, by bending the knees with the feet flat on the bed, raises the buttocks. For extra tension, you can use your arms to lift your head and shoulders as well. If you find it tiring you can support yourself with a cushion or two under the buttocks. Throw your head right back to increase the sense of offering the genitals.

Supta Vajrasana – the kneeling pose

This is a position that in yoga requires you to keep your thighs together, but for *maithuna* yoga or sexual yoga you should obviously keep them well apart. Kneel on the bed, place your hands on the bed behind you and lean back as far as possible. To increase the tension even more and, indeed, do the position properly, carry on until your head and back touch the bed. But if you can't manage it, just go as far as you can. Your partner lays or kneels between your thighs and, as a result of the tension along the inner thighs, you'll enjoy some powerful sensations.

As a variation you can kneel astride your partner's chest and while he or she provides oral sex you can lean back and use your fingers on your partner's genitals.

Summary

- In the *Kama Sutra*, use of the fingers, lips and tongue is always 'foreplay' and not an end in itself.
- A man never succeeds with a woman 'without a great deal of talking'.
- The *Kama Sutra* describes many different ways of embracing, culminating in the embrace of the *jaghana*.
- There are at least half a dozen different ways of kissing.
- Kissing can be made into a game with wagers and forfeits for the loser.
- Foreplay creates lubrication but it's always a good idea to have something extra.
- Oral sex or *auparishtaka* was a technique disapproved of by many ancient Hindus.
- The *Kama Sutra* describes eight different ways of performing fellatio.
- For the sake of great cunnilingus, courtesans would abandon men 'possessed of good qualities'.
- Vatsyayana didn't specifically mention the clitoris.
- Vatsyayana says a man should make his fingers into the form of an elephant's trunk to stimulate the *yoni*.
- The position known as the 'congress of a crow' is for simultaneous oral sex.

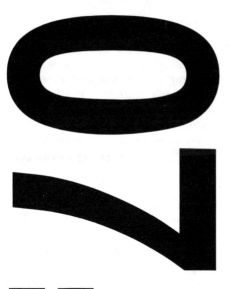

07 pleasure and pain

In this chapter you will learn:
- how pleasure and pain are linked
- how pretend quarrels, scratching, biting and slapping can be used in foreplay
- how moans, groans and 'coarse' words increase excitement.

Sexual intercourse can be compared to a quarrel, on account of the contrarieties of love and its tendency to dispute ... During the excitement, when the woman is not accustomed to striking, she continually utters words expressive of prohibition, sufficiency, or desire of liberation, as well as the words 'father', 'mother', intermingled with the sighing, weeping and thundering sound.

The *Kama Sutra*

The *Kama Sutra* devotes even more space to quarrelling and to scratching, biting and slapping than it does to sexual positions. Vatsyayana knew very well what scientists today have proven beyond doubt, that stress enhances sexual arousal, which is no doubt why sex is sometimes referred to as 'a bit of slap and tickle'.

It's all to do with evolution – or, more accurately, the lack of it. We still have as one of the most primitive parts of our brains the same so-called limbic system that many animals have. It handles our most basic drives. So it's not altogether surprising if we sometimes feel like biting and scratching when we're having sex, because that's what a lot of mammals do.

But it's important to keep well within the bounds of love play and not cause real pain. Vatsyayana's solution, very much in keeping with the Indian outlook, was to ritualize these things and lay down a set of rules. He even went so far as to specify how mock quarrels should be conducted.

All of this works because the body's hormonal response to stress is very similar to its hormonal response to sex. What's more, intense stimulation of the skin increases the blood supply, making the skin far more sensitive.

Sexual intercourse, says Vatsyayana, can be compared to a quarrel. It's a concept that seems to have appealed very much to the people of his time.

The quarrel

In the West we have the expression 'kiss and make up'. In other words, the idea that you have an argument but that the making up afterwards is worth it.

In Vatsyayana's India quarrels were spectacular and theatrical: 'The woman cries, becomes angry, tosses her hair about, strikes her lover, falls from her bed or seat and, casting aside her garlands and ornaments, throws herself down on the ground.'

The man should then try to placate her, lifting her up and carrying her to the bed. But this is not yet enough. The woman should now proceed to the door, 'having kicked him once, twice, or thrice on his arms, head, bosom, or back'. Only when she's sure her partner's apologies have 'reached their utmost' should she calm down.

It's a piece of pure opera that probably has little appeal to most Western couples, but you might like to try adapting it to suit you and see what happens.

Have a go: Chasing

Remember, this is a mock quarrel and not the real thing, so don't pick on something that's a significant issue between you. The idea is simply to create some excitement and get the blood pumping.

- If your man is always watching sport on TV, for example, you could stand in front of the screen and complain that he's more interested in watching football than a real woman.
- Tell your partner she or he has been very naughty and is going to get a good spanking.
- Snatch something of your partner's and run off with it for a game of chase me, catch me.
- Take your knickers off, throw them at your partner and run for it. (For some reason this never seems to work so well when a man does it.)
- Let's say you're hosing the garden or washing the car on a nice, sunny day and some of the water 'accidentally' makes your partner's clothes wet.

Once you've chased around and caught one another you can move onto the next stage.

Getting physical

The *Kama Sutra* recommends three different ways of inflicting a little pain:

- pressing, marking or scratching with the nails
- biting
- striking.

Scratching

According to the *Kama Sutra*, the use of the nails is for those who are 'intensely passionate'. With his usual precision Vatsyayana lists eight different marks the nails can leave on the body. Rather more useful is his advice that the initial touch should be so light that 'only the hair on the body becomes erect'. But the nails were also used to leave semi-permanent marks, especially if one of the lovers was going away for a time. He quotes a saying that the love of a woman who sees the marks of nails 'on the private parts of her body, even though they are old and almost worn out, becomes again fresh and new'.

Biting

Just as there are eight ways with nails so there are eight kinds of bites, ranging from a bite that leaves the skin a little red right up to biting that leaves rows of teeth marks. According to the *Kama Sutra*, if a man bites a woman she should bite him back – and harder.

Striking

Vatsyayana proposes four different ways of striking – with the back of the hand, with the fingers slightly contracted, with the fist and with the open palm. He even gives instructions for the sounds the person being struck should make, including thundering sounds, cooing sounds and noises like a parrot, a bee and a flamingo. Once again, it's all part of the rituals the ancient Hindus enjoyed so much.

'Blows with the fist should be given on the back of the woman, while she is sitting on the lap of the man,' Vatsyayana advises. She should then hit him in return, meanwhile abusing him 'as if she were angry'.

Conscious of the potential hazards, Vatsyayana cites the King of the Panchalas who killed the courtesan Madhavasena by accident: 'A horse having once attained the fifth degree of motion,' he warns, 'goes on with blind speed, regardless of pits, ditches and posts in his way; and in the same manner a loving pair become blind with passion in the heat of congress, and go on with great impetuosity, paying not the least regard to excess.'

Have a go: But how hard is hard?

Nowadays, with the newspapers continually full of stories about domestic and other violence, many of us are so repelled by it that the idea of deliberately hurting our partners even a tiny bit is abhorrent. And quite right too. But there is a level of sensation that lies somewhere between caressing and actual pain that is nevertheless both arousing and enjoyable. If we're too timid in our lovemaking we'll never experience it.

The first thing to do is to try out Vatsyayana's 'scratching', 'biting' and 'striking' on yourself. Your partner should do the same. Go through the techniques one by one gradually applying more and more force. Find out which parts of the body are the most sensitive. Something that is barely perceptible in one location may actually cause real pain in another.

Now try things out with your partner, but not yet in a sexual situation (in which you might get carried away). Just run through the techniques on different parts of one another's bodies. You'll probably feel quite silly doing it. The whole point, of course, is to tell your partner when you can't feel something at all and when, at the other extreme, something really hurts.

When you've completed your homework you can get down to real sex. A word of warning, mostly for women. Never take part in this sort of love play if you're not completely sure of your partner. Secondly, never do it if you believe your partner deep down is angry with you or harbouring some unspoken resentments. If sex extinguishes normal restraint you could end up getting seriously hurt.

Once again, you might feel rather silly at first using Vatsyayana's techniques. You'll probably have to keep encouraging and reassuring one another. 'No, it didn't hurt. Really. Try it a bit harder.' But if you're doing it right you'll soon find you're reaching a degree of arousal all over your body that you've previously experienced only in your genital area (this applies especially to men).

The idea of pain leading to pleasure is not confined to the *Kama Sutra*, of course. As we've seen, many Victorian brothels had their 'dungeons', and if you examine catalogues of sex toys you'll often find things like whips and 'paddles', which are used for spanking.

Bondage

Bondage – tying your partner up – isn't mentioned in the *Kama Sutra*, but as it's closely linked with pleasure and pain in most people's minds I'm going to say a little bit about it.

In fact, there's no reason at all that bondage has to involve even the tiniest amount of pain. Most couples don't use it that way. What bondage is really all about is:

- being the focus of attention
- being absolved of any guilt for what happens.

A whole range of bondage accessories is available in sex shops or on the internet, but, to start with, you can simply use things that are to hand.

First a word of caution. Never allow yourself to be tied up by someone you don't know extremely well. Even a person you've lived with for quite a while can exhibit behaviour you never dreamed of. Don't permit any restraints initially that can't, if necessary, be undone or broken by you. If you both enjoy yourselves and all is well you can move onto something stronger later on.

Have a go: light bondage

- Love play: raise your partner's arms so they're stretched out along the pillow or bed behind and pin them there.
- Men: when undressing your partner in bed, pull her underwear down to her knees or ankles and leave it there. If she's agreeable and flexible enough, with her underwear around her knees she could pull her legs back and you could slip the gusset behind her head. If she's less flexible (or has flimsy underwear) you can achieve the same effect with a scarf.
- Handcuffs: use cheap plastic ones that can be broken easily. Only use metal ones if you're totally confident. Either of you could have your arms handcuffed behind your back, for example. For a laugh, you could both wear handcuffs and see if you can manage to make love at all.

Have a go: medium bondage

One of you should be tied, spread-eagled, to the bed. Of course you need to have a suitable bed. But being tied up is only the start. The person who isn't tied up still has to do something.

- Give your partner your full attention, without thinking about your own satisfaction. Perform a striptease; masturbate; bring your body close but not close enough to touch; arouse him/her a little then go away leaving your partner in a state of delicious anticipation.

- Surprise your partner – but make sure it's a nice surprise. It can increase the excitement considerably to cover your partner's eyes with a blindfold. He or she won't then know what you're about to do. Make sure it's something nice. Describe it first: 'I'm going to play with myself' or 'I'm going to bite your nipples.'

- Try stimulating your partner's skin with different things – feathers, a brush, ice, massage oil, whatever you can think of.

- Push the boundaries further than they've been pushed before – but only a little further. If you know your partner feels guilty about stimulation of the anal area, for example, then this could be the moment to do it.

- Bondage often goes hand in hand with a certain style of dressing up for sex. Rubber dresses and underwear are popular.

The sounds of sex

Vatsyayana gives very precise instructions for the sounds someone should make when they've been struck. They seem rather comical at first, and, indeed, the distinction between 'phut' and 'phat' is something that is now lost to us. 'Phat', he explains, is the sound of a bamboo being split, while 'phut' is the sound of something falling into water.

What we can relate to rather more easily are 'cooing', 'sighing' and 'weeping' sounds, and the woman using words 'expressive of prohibition, sufficiency, or desire of liberation', as well as the words 'father' and 'mother'.

In the West, quite a lot of couples neither talk nor make any sound at all while having sex. But this was clearly not the Indian way. In fact, noises are some of the best aphrodisiacs that exist.

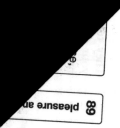

when your partner is getting excited. They tell
hen you're getting excited. And, somehow, they
more immediately into play.

rrassed about the concept and don't believe that
ry it while masturbating. You'll find you become
quickly and more powerfully if you deliberately
an.

Love talk

However, there's no need to leave sounds at just a series of
moans and exclamations. Words are even more powerful than
noises. Nothing excites a partner as much as words assembled
in the right combination. Don't worry, you don't need to be a
poet. The *Kama Sutra* says lovers should 'talk suggestively of
things which would be considered as coarse, or not to be
mentioned generally in society'. In other words, what we'd
nowadays call 'talking dirty'.

So what exactly *do* you say? At the beginning of an encounter it
isn't always easy, or appropriate, to get too 'dirty'. So first of all
just let your partner know if he or she is doing the right thing:
'That's exactly the right place'. 'A bit lower'. 'Faster'. Or
whatever. Compliment your partner when it's good rather than
criticize when it's bad: 'The pressure you used just then was
perfect.'

Secondly, you need to be sure *you're* doing the right thing.
'Here?' 'Faster?' 'Slower?' And so on. Admittedly, these kinds of
questions would get a bit tedious if you had to ask them every
time, but you won't. Next time you'll know.

Once you've both got a bit excited you can get 'dirtier'. Don't
use the dictionary words. Just say whatever comes into your
head. Put words to your feelings. Obviously, try not to use
words you know your partner objects to. On the other hand,
during the excitement, different standards apply.

If nothing immediately comes into your head, here are some
suggestions:

- Describe how excited your partner is making you.
- Describe what you're going to do to your partner.
- Tell your partner how you want him/her to lie or sit or kneel
  or whatever.
- Say what it is about your partner that turns you on.

- Tell your partner what you want him/her to do to you.
- Describe the stage of excitement you've reached.

As your excitement grows your words will become less and less intelligible. They'll be gasped out. And, finally, shrieked.

Fantasy

Fantasy is probably the ultimate turn-on. Vatsyayana's 'coarse' talk taken to its most powerful level.

If you haven't yet discovered this for yourself, masturbate in your normal way without fantasy. After a while, continue masturbating while visualizing, for example, that you're a maharajah in your harem. Or a maharani in the harem into which your secret lover has been smuggled. Whatever turns you on. Almost immediately you'll notice an increase in your excitement.

Fantasizing while masturbating is wonderful. You don't have to worry about upsetting a partner. You don't have to worry about being thought weird. There's just you and your imagination. You can be with any film star you choose, any friend or acquaintance, any number of people, in any place, doing anything you want.

Use props if you like. Men often like to use their partners' underwear to help them visualize that she's actually there.

Now say something out loud, as if, for example, addressing someone in your fantasy. Be as 'dirty' as you wish. Perhaps say something you've never dared to say before. You'll probably orgasm straight away, or be very close to doing so.

You might consider that sexual fantasies are fine for masturbation but unhealthy with a partner. The *Kama Sutra* talks of a kind of fantasy called the 'congress of transferred love'. It's when you make love while fantasizing that your partner is someone else that you'd prefer to be with. Now that *is* unhealthy. But there are other kinds of fantasy that you can share together. These kinds of fantasies can be extremely positive. Once you start sharing fantasies you're laying bare your partner's mind and soul. You're going deeper and getting more intimate than ever before.

Fantasies can:

- raise the level of excitement

- shortcut arousal
- go straight to the relevant parts of the brain
- reveal things about your partner you never knew before
- increase the sense of intimacy between you
- introduce ideas you *can* go on to use in reality if you wish.

At one end of the spectrum, you might simply introduce a fantasy about something you'd like to do together but have never dared mention before. During the excitement of sex, for example, you might 'confess' you once had a dream about licking and sucking your partner's *lingam* or *yoni* and that in this dream your partner was driven wild. At the other end of the spectrum might come a totally impossible fantasy involving, say, a harem of a hundred women – or men.

The *Kama Sutra* itself provides plenty of fantasy material for both men and women:

- The threesome: 'When a man enjoys two women at the same time, both of whom love him equally, it is called the "united congress".'
- Lesbianism: 'The women of the royal harem cannot see or meet any men … For this reason, among themselves they give pleasure to each other in various ways as now described. Having dressed … like men, they accomplish their object with bulbs, roots and fruits having the form of the *lingam*.'
- The secret lover: 'By means of their female attendants the ladies of the royal harem generally get men into their apartments in the disguise or dress of women.'
- The orgy: 'The entrance of young men into harems, and their exit from them, generally takes place when things are being brought into the palace … A young man who enjoys all of them, and who is common to them all, can continue enjoying his union with them so long as it is kept quiet …'

Have a go

- Try to find out what your partner's sexual fantasies are. He or she is almost certain to have them. Take note of your partner's favourite books, TV programmes, films and actors.
- Fantasies can blow your mind but they can also blow up your relationship if you start on a subject your partner is frightened about, so proceed cautiously.
- Once you think you know the right subject, just hint at it during sex and see if your partner responds. If he/she doesn't take up

> the idea, don't press it. Try again another day after the concept has had time to sink in.
> - If your partner does respond, take turns to progress the story, prompting one another and carrying on the narrative.
> - As always, proceed slowly. Introduce new ideas one small step at a time.
> - You'll know you're on the right track if your partner's lovemaking becomes more frantic.

It sometimes happens that the one to introduce fantasy into lovemaking is then shocked by a partner's response. Suddenly, you could be confronted by ideas you weren't expecting and find difficult to deal with. You may feel that by unlocking these fantasies you've encouraged behaviour that, in the real world, would be devastating to you. Relax. This is unlikely to be the case. Remember that your partner has always had these fantasies. The only difference is that now you know about them.

In fact, your partner will feel relieved and probably even exhilarated that his or her fantasies are in the open. Better sex is all about the freedom to be yourself in the presence of another person. By expressing your innermost thoughts and feelings, and allowing your partner to do the same, you're taking sex to its highest level.

Introducing fantasy is like a direct line into the brain. It can cause arousal far faster than any physical technique. Once you're 'up there' you don't necessarily have to continue the fantasy any further. Nor should you use fantasy every time. Treat it like other techniques – not something to be used repetitively but a part of the range of things you can do.

Summary

- A *little* mental and physical stress can enhance sexual pleasure.
- The *Kama Sutra* recommends pretend quarrels, but you may simply prefer a game of 'chase me, catch me'.
- When you've caught one another, scratching, biting and slapping can all increase physical arousal.
- Test your techniques on yourself first, to make sure they don't hurt too much.
- When you introduce the techniques with your partner, check to make sure the level is right.

- You can extend the concept with bondage if you wish.
- Make plenty of noise during sex – it's a turn on for both of you.
- The *Kama Sutra* says you should 'talk suggestively' about things that are 'coarse'.
- Avoid the private fantasy the *Kama Sutra* calls the 'congress of transferred love', but share fantasies together.

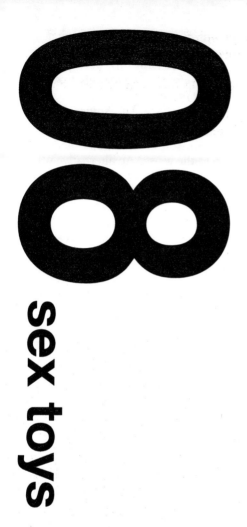

08

sex toys

In this chapter you will learn:
- what sex toys existed at the time of the *Kama Sutra*
- which sex toys work best
- what methods of enlarging the penis work best.

When a man wishes to enlarge his lingam, he should rub it with the bristles of certain insects that live in trees, and then, after rubbing it for ten nights with oils, he should again rub it with the bristles as before. By continuing to do this a swelling will be gradually produced ...

The *Kama Sutra*

'The *kantuka* or *jalaka*,' Vatsyayana wrote, 'is a tube ... outwardly rough and studded with soft globules, and made to fit the size of the *yoni*, and tied to the waist.' An alternative was the 'tubular stalk of the bottle gourd'. This is what we would nowadays call a 'strap-on'. That's to say, a dildo attached to a harness. If you thought sex toys were a modern invention you're in for a surprise.

Vatsyayana didn't specify when to employ the *kantuka* except to say it could be used in place of the *lingam*, presumably, as nowadays, by a man suffering from premature ejaculation, impotence, an unusually small penis or, simply, fatigue. The ancient Hindus also experimented with various kinds of 'cock cages' to increase stimulation and the depth of penetration, as well as penis piercings and various concoctions to enlarge the penis, stiffen the penis, enlarge or contract the vagina, increase desire and, not surprisingly, make women fall in love. Many of these things would be perfectly recognizable to us today.

In Vatsyayana's time, men and women would have had to prepare their own toys and elixirs. Nowadays, all you have to do is go to your nearest sex shop.

Shopping for sex toys

Even chemists have now begun to sell sex toys, but for a full range you really need to go to a sex shop. It's an interesting test of how you really feel about sex. Take a look at the following two groups of statements. Which are closest to your own feelings, the first group or the second?

Group 1:

- I park my car some way off in case anybody recognizes it.
- I wear dark glasses.
- I always pay cash just in case my bank or credit card company should know I've been in a sex shop.
- I come out without having bought what I really wanted.

Group 2:

- I don't mind who sees me go into the sex shop.
- I discuss the merits of the various products with the sales assistant.
- I have a good laugh about some of the toys.
- I like to try out the latest ideas and designs.

If the first group of statements most closely represents your outlook then you have some work to do on your attitudes. If you're more in line with the second group then you're ready to take the *Kama Sutra*'s advice on *apadravyas* or 'apparatus'.

Ideally, visit the sex shop as a couple. Make it a bit of an occasion. If you've never been before, fight the impulse to turn and flee the moment you step through the door. Some things will surprise you, some will make you laugh, some will probably evoke a 'yuk', and some you may end up buying. You'll probably discover things about one another's sexual feelings that you never knew before.

If there isn't a convenient sex shop, or you're too embarrassed to go in, take a look on the internet (see 'Taking it further'). With hundreds of online suppliers to choose from you're obviously going to have a much bigger choice than one shop can provide. But you're not going to be able to try your toys out the same day.

Dildos

A dildo is an artificial *lingam* which does nothing on its own. In order to create an effect, the woman herself or her partner has to move it. Dildos don't feature much in Indian erotic art but ancient Chinese erotic paintings often show women with dildos strapped to their feet. That way they could manipulate the dildo while keeping their hands free for other kinds of stimulation.

The *Kama Sutra* says a man should use a dildo if he is unable to satisfy a woman. They should be made of 'gold, silver, copper, iron, ivory, buffalo's horn, various kinds of wood, tin or lead'.

Since the invention of the vibrator, dildos might seem to be redundant. And yet dildos are now having a renaissance, thanks not to any of those materials but to glass. Normally, in fact, pyrex. With strands of colour woven into them they have a beauty that plastic dildos don't and some are so elegant they even come with stands so they can be displayed beside the bed.

The 'designer' ones can cost even more than a pair of designer jeans but, fortunately, there are less expensive models as well.

But why buy one when you could have a vibrator? The answer is that the G-spot responds far more to pressure than it does to vibration. (If you don't know how to find the G-spot, take a look at Chapter 11.) What's more, glass has very particular qualities. It can be put in the fridge for a cool sensation, or into a mug of warm water. Being incredibly smooth, little or no lubrication is required. And being non-porous, glass is very hygienic – a glass dildo can even be put in the dishwasher.

Have a go: Women

- Look for a dildo that has a large round head or, even better, a head with marbles. An extra protuberance for the clitoris is a good idea.
- If you like the idea of glass but also want vibrations, there are models with a hole into which a vibrating 'bullet' can be inserted. Glass transmits the vibrations extremely well, which gives you the best of both worlds.
- Wash your dildo before using it.
- Excite yourself in your normal way, apply a little lubricant to the dildo and insert it into your *yoni*.
- Compare the effect of moving it in and out with the effect of simply squeezing your PC muscle to press it against your G-spot. (If you can't remember about the PC muscle, take a look again at Chapter 04.)

Have a go: Men

- Look for a dildo that's specially shaped to stimulate the prostate gland. (If you don't know how to locate the prostate, see Chapter 11.)
- Wash your dildo before using it.
- Excite yourself in your normal way, apply a generous amount of lubricant to the dildo and slowly and gently ease it into your rectum.
- Squeeze your PC muscle to press the dildo against your prostate gland. (If you can't remember about the PC muscle, take a look again at Chapter 04; for more on anal techniques, see Chapter 11.)

Vibrators

Vibrators are dildos that have a little motor inside them to make them vibrate. If you haven't tried one, get one immediately. They sell in their millions and there's absolutely nothing 'kinky' about them at all. Women use them on their own, men use them on their own and couples use them together.

The traditional vibrator is approximately the size and shape of a *lingam*, either in a realistic skin colour or in anything from white to fluorescent orange. More recently other 'non-penis' designs have been introduced because, in fact, most women prefer the vibrations on or close to the clitoris, not in the *yoni*. You'll also have to decide between soft and hard models. Most people opt for a soft vibrator, initially, but, in fact, it's the hard designs that deliver the most intense vibrations.

Women who have never had an orgasm often experience their first one with a vibrator. The less orgasmic a woman is, the more powerful the vibrator needs to be. If you really have a problem reaching orgasm you might like to consider a mains-powered model. They can also double as body massagers. But women who are normally orgasmic tend to find them too powerful – they can quickly cause numbness rather than ecstasy.

Have a go

- Wash your vibrator before using it (if it's mains-powered, follow the cleaning instructions).

- If you're on your own, experiment with the vibrator all over your body, paying particular attention to your neck, breasts, nipples and, of course, vulva.

- You'll almost certainly find the most effective technique is to apply the tip of the vibrator on or close to the clitoris, depending on how sensitive you are.

- Apply some lubricant and see what happens when you slide the vibrator in and out of your *yoni*.

- Press the vibrator against your G-spot. (If you don't know how to find the G-spot, take a look at Chapter 11.)

- If you're with your partner, don't let him plunge the vibrator in and out of your *yoni*; it probably won't feel particularly good and may even hurt.

- The best thing with a partner is to let him watch you masturbate with the vibrator; most men find it very exciting.

- During intercourse the vibrator can still be used. Either of you can play it on your clitoris, for example, or while you're lying flat on the bed, face down, the vibrator can be slipped underneath, against your vulva.

Anal vibrators

Vibrators specially designed for the *payau* (anus) and rectum are usually narrower than standard models but with a wide base so they can't accidentally slip all the way in. If you've never used one before, start with something small; if you enjoy it you can work up to a larger size. For men there are models with a tip angled specifically for the prostate gland.

There's disagreement between translators over the extent to which the *Kama Sutra* describes anal sex. Most scholars interpret 'women acting the part of a man' simply to mean women getting on top. Others, particularly Daniélou, believe Vatsyayana was talking about women using dildos on their men.

Whoever is right, there are two particularly exciting ways of using anal vibrators during intercourse:

- A man can slide one into his partner's rectum during intercourse, so you can *both* feel the sensations.
- A man can insert one into his own rectum during intercourse, to intensify his personal stimulation.

There's more on *adhorata* (anal sex) in Chapter 11.

Specialist vibrators

The little electric motors that cause the vibrations are every month being installed into all kinds of fantastic new devices and shapes.

There are *lingam*-shaped vibrators that also make circling movements. There are vibrators for the *yoni* that also have protrusions for the clitoris. And there are vibrators designed specifically for the G-spot. These models have a tip that's curved or even at right-angles to the body of the toy. Again, it's far easier for the woman to find the right spot herself than for her partner to do it (because he won't be getting any direct feedback as he would with his finger).

Then there are double vibrators that stimulate both the vagina and the anus/rectum simultaneously, often with a special protrusion for the clitoris as well. A different kind of double vibrator has a *lingam* pointing in each direction. These are aimed principally at lesbians but heterosexual couples can also use them, the woman having one end in her *yoni* while the man has the other in his *payau*.

Harnesses and strap-ons exist which very much allow a woman to act 'the part of a man'. Again, these can be used by lesbians but also by heterosexual couples who want to switch roles. The man can feel what it's like to be penetrated (in the rectum) and the woman can get some idea of what it's like to do the penetrating in exactly the way a man does it.

Yet another category can be worn by a woman. The vibrator is incorporated into a G-string and presses against the clitoris, or simply slides into a pair of panties. Some can even be operated by remote control, which can make for a bit of fun at, say, a boring business meeting or dinner party. You can even get vibrators to attach to mobile phones – so you're always pleased when your partner phones – and to your iPod to give you orgasms in time to music.

For clitoral stimulators worn on the *lingam*, see below.

Vibrators for men

An ordinary vibrator can be used by a woman on a man or by a man on himself. Simply hold the vibrator against the penis. Try different spots to see what happens.

But there are vibrators specially designed for men to wear on their penises (stimulating both of you at the same time) as well as vibrators in the form of *yonis* (stimulating only the man).

The vibrating cock ring is something the man wears around the base of his penis so that, during intercourse, it presses against the clitoris. The man feels the vibrations along his penis and, as a result, the woman not only feels them on her clitoris but also inside her vagina. They used to be rather cumbersome affairs with wires that got in the way, but now there's a new generation powered by internal watch batteries. These are good fun for everyone but especially for men who have a problem keeping their erections.

Naturally, some designers have taken the concept even further and added things like anal probes and anal beads which vibrate inside the rectum at the same time.

A word of caution about cock rings that constrict the penis in order to prevent the blood flowing out (and therefore maintain an erection). *They can do damage.* Never take any risks with your penis.

Artificial *yonis* are generally for men to use on their own but there's no reason you shouldn't masturbate together, each using your favourite toy. What's more, this could be the solution for a man who needs a lot of stimulation to maintain an erection. Nowadays these *yonis* are made of materials that have an amazingly natural feel. One of the best is Cyberskin but there are new materials coming along all the time. You can even buy a *yoni* modelled on your favourite porn star. What these *yonis* can't do is stretch like the real thing, so you'll need to measure the length and circumference of your erect penis and then look for a model to fit.

Toys and techniques for penis enlargement

Rubbing the penis with insect bristles is just the start of one of Vatsyayana's recipes for enlarging the *lingam*. The next stage was to lie on a cot with a hole in it so that the *lingam* would hang down. The resultant swelling, known as *suka*, was said to be for life.

But before we look any further at Vatsyayana's ideas, let's just ask the question that obviously goes back at least two thousand years: does size matter? Vatsyayana clearly thought it did: 'Man is divided into three classes: the hare men, the bull man, and the horse man, according to the size of his *lingam*. Woman also, according to the depth of her *yoni* is either a female deer, a mare, or a female elephant ... There are, then, nine kinds of union according to dimensions. Among all these, equal unions are the best.'

In his commentary, Yashodhara says the hare man is six fingers, the bull man nine fingers and the horse man 12 fingers, but there's some disagreement as to what constitutes the width of a finger. Burton, possibly having small hands, calculated that *lingams* were from 7.5cm to 15cm. Other commentators say from 11cm to 22cm. Nowadays the average is said to be about 14cm in erection, but nobody really knows.

Yashodhara agreed that size mattered, quoting a verse to the effect that women would never grow very fond of a man with a small penis, no matter how much effort he made.

In Western society, women have not yet become paranoid about *their* size, but Vatsyayana makes a sensible point when he discusses male dimensions in relation to female dimensions. Here's why size *doesn't* matter:

- The average woman, who has never had children, has a *yoni* that is just 7.5cm long and 2cm in diameter. When excited it becomes about 10cm long.
- Only the outer third of the vagina is very sensitive, amounting to little more than 2.5cm.
- So even the smallest *lingam* can excite any *yoni*.
- The *yoni* has the ability to stretch considerably to accommodate a 'horse man' (but the woman's partner needs to take care not to bump against an ovary).
- So even the largest *lingam* can fit any *yoni*.
- Different positions can vary the apparent depth and width of the *yoni* as well as the depth of penetration (as we'll see in Chapters 09 and 10)

Among a *lingam's* physical attributes, then, size is of minor importance. Far more significant are sensitivity and the ability to maintain an erect state. Those are the things that influence a couple's pleasure.

So now let's return to the *Kama Sutra's* secret recipes. No doubt there are many ways of making a penis swollen, but a *lingam* that is truly enlarged in erection is a different matter. Is there any science behind the instruction to massage the *lingam* in oil in which watermelon, aubergine, buffalo butter, the castor oil plant and various other things had been boiled?

In fact, there probably isn't anything in the ingredients so much as in the massage. The penis, you see, is supported by connective ligaments. These are the things that are cut in surgical penis enlargement, but they can also be stretched. Either way, although the penis remains the same length, it can then extend further away from the body.

Stretching is something that has to be done at least three times a week and preferably every day. In addition to lengthening the ligaments it can also lengthen the blood spaces inside the *lingam* itself. When those spaces fill with blood, as they do in erection, so the penis is longer.

Well, that's the theory. Is there any proof? In fact, there is some. In 1975, Dr Brian Richards carried out experiments with 64 men (a number that would have appealed to Vatsyayana). Of those, half were a control. Of the half that were actually following the enlargement technique, two dropped out and two gained nothing. The remaining 28 gained up to 3.5cm in length and up to 3cm in girth in the space of just three months. That was a success rate of 87.5 per cent.

So how do you go about this stretching? The men in Dr Richards' trial were actually using vacuum pumps. In sex shops you'll also see weights for hanging on your penis, rather like Vatsyayana's technique of hanging the penis through a hole in the bed. And there are even devices to stretch the scrotum so that the testicles hang lower and are more visible. But those methods have risks. Remember: a small penis is better than a penis that doesn't work. Don't take any chances.

Have a go: penis massage

Massage is a safe method, as long as it's done correctly and gently. Never use a lot of force, otherwise you might damage the walls of the blood vessels. Here's how to do it safely:

- Make sure your penis is warm. If it's not, take a bath or shower or wrap it in a flannel soaked in hot water.
- Apply a little evening primrose oil to your penis and testicles.
- Place your two thumbs on top of your penis at the very base.
- Place the forefingers and middle fingers on the underside of the penis, leaving a little space for the urethra (the tube through which you urinate and ejaculate).
- Now, very slowly and gently move your fingers towards the glans, stretching out the penis as you go.
- When you reach the tip, stretch your penis out gently by tugging the foreskin (if you have one). You'll see the tendons at the base being pulled taut.
- Repeat for up to 20 minutes.
- Whenever you get an erection, stop and let it subside.
- Finish off by gently massaging your testicles.

Even if your penis doesn't become significantly larger, a regular massage, properly done, can only be a good thing.

Piercing the *lingam* was yet another technique described in the *Kama Sutra* and still used in parts of Asia today. Various things were then attached, with the aim of increasing stimulation to the *yoni* – not a technique that can be recommended. But you can safely get something of the same effect using special condoms with twiddly bits, 'cock cages' that go over the erect penis to give it a 'knobbly' feel, and toys that fit over the glans and shaft of the penis. Alternatively, try slipping love balls into your partner's *yoni* and then – gently – making love.

Summary

- The ancient Hindus had dildos, 'cock cages' and other sex toys.
- Don't be embarrassed about going into sex shops but, if you are, or there's no convenient sex shop, you can get everything you want on the internet.
- Dildos might seem redundant but they're particularly good for the G-spot.
- Vibrators should be used by all couples; they're particularly good for women who don't orgasm easily.
- Anal vibrators can increase the power of orgasm for both of you.
- Vibrators worn on the *lingam* can help a man maintain his erection, as well as provide extra stimulation to the *yoni* and clitoris.
- Special vibrators in the form of *yonis* exist for men.
- Penis enlargement devices carry risks but massage can be a safe alternative.
- According to the *Kama Sutra*, intercourse is best when a couple are of 'equal size' but, in reality, size doesn't matter.

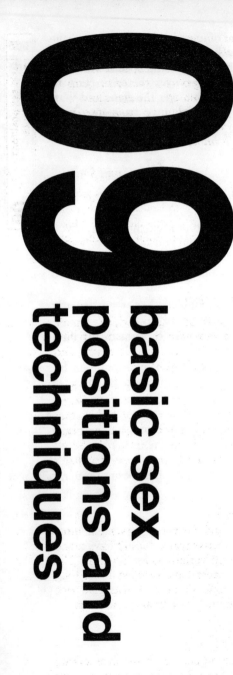

09

basic sex positions and techniques

In this chapter you will learn:
- ways of moving
- reasons for using a variety of positions
- the easiest *real* positions of the *Kama Sutra*.

Such passionate actions and amorous gesticulations or movements, which arise on the spur of the moment, and during sexual intercourse, cannot be defined, and are as irregular as dreams. A horse having once attained the fifth degree of motion goes on with blind speed, regardless of pits, ditches, and posts in his way; and in the same manner a loving pair become blind with passion in the heat of congress, and go on with great impetuosity, paying not the least regard to excess.

The *Kama Sutra*

Most positions of the *Kama Sutra* aren't as difficult as people imagine. And even if you don't manage to pull all of them off, you'll certainly have a lot of fun trying. In this chapter we look at the easier ones, together with ways of moving. In the next chapter we'll look at the really tricky ones.

Ways of moving for men

The *Kama Sutra* says that, 'if a male be long-timed, the female loves him the more, but if he be short-timed she is dissatisfied with him … it takes a long time to allay a woman's desire, and during this time she is enjoying great pleasure …'

One of the keys to being 'long-timed' is for a man to alternate highly stimulating movements with less stimulating movements. It's also the way to maintain 'great pleasure' for his partner because, as all women know, the vulva and the vagina can begin to feel numb if the same stimulation is given constantly. So all nine ways of moving described by the *Kama Sutra* are worth trying out.

Moving the organ forward

This is the standard backwards and forwards movement most couples use most of the time, and Vatsyayana doesn't have much to say about it. But lots of different variations are possible. The Chinese Taoist tradition, which must have reached India long before, suggests, for example, nine shallow thrusts and one deep, five shallow and one deep, one shallow and one deep.

Churning

A simple yet highly effective technique, which involves taking hold of the base of the *lingam* in your fist. Obviously you won't now be able to plunge it in to its full length, but that doesn't really matter because the most sensitive part of the vagina, as we've already seen, is the outer third. Now move your *lingam* in a circling motion, round and round inside the entrance to the *yoni*. Apply a little extra pressure each time you pass the roof of the vagina because that's where the famous G-spot is located (see Chapter 11).

As a refinement you can let your knuckles bump against the clitoris while you churn. Alternatively, you can hold your *lingam* with your thumb at the top (nail trimmed short) so the pad of your thumb rubs against the clitoris all the time that you're churning.

Churning is also something a man can do by moving his hips. This allows deeper penetration, since the hand isn't in the way, but it's not easy to keep the movement up for very long.

Piercing and rubbing

The translations just don't agree about piercing and rubbing, but essentially we're concerned here about angling the *lingam* downwards to stimulate the floor of the *yoni* (and therefore the clitoris at the same time) and angling it up to stimulate the roof of the *yoni* (and therefore the G-spot at the same time). You can switch from one to the other by changing the angle of your hips, which will make your lingam sort of 'wave' inside the *yoni*.

Pressing

All translations seem to agree on pressing. It simply means pushing the penis right in and keeping it there. However, don't do this until the woman is fully relaxed and lubricated. As a variation, the man (without moving the *lingam* inside the *yoni*) can grind himself a little against the woman's vulva so as to stimulate her clitoris, or simply push intermittently against her. This can be a useful technique for prolonged intercourse because it provides very little stimulation to the man.

Giving a blow

Once again, all translations are clear that giving a blow involves the man withdrawing completely then plunging back in from a short distance. It can be very exciting from the psychological as well as the physical point of view: psychologically, because the moment of penetration is full of significance for both women and men; physically, because the entrance to the *yoni* is extremely sensitive and tighter than the part further in. So withdrawing and re-entering time after time can be pretty mind-blowing for both of you.

It's a technique to use when the vagina is thoroughly excited, the lips pulled back and the entrance open. But, even so, don't withdraw more than 5cm or you might miss your target and bang painfully against the clitoris. Try varying the length of time you withdraw. It could be for just a second, five seconds or even 15 seconds.

The blow of a boar and the blow of a bull

Apparently, a boar thrusts to one side of the vagina only while a bull thrusts alternately against one side and then the other.

Sporting of a sparrow

This is the movement intended to bring lovemaking to a climax and which Vatsyayana likens to the pecking of a bird. When the woman is close to orgasm, the man makes a series of quick thrusts, some shallow, some deep, until she comes.

Ways of moving for women

The *Kama Sutra* says a woman 'should do in return the same actions which he used to do before', and she should tell her partner: 'I was laid down by you, and fatigued with hard congress; I shall now therefore lay you down in return.'

Here, then, are some of the things a woman can do:

- Take hold of the base of your partner's *lingam* in your fist and experiment with different ways of moving it. Try rubbing the glans against your clitoris or circling it inside the entrance to your *yoni*. In one of the woman-on-top-positions you can also move up and down on it, letting your clitoris bump against your hand.

- In one of the woman-on-top-positions, try sliding up and down the full length of the *lingam*. Try short movements. Try withdrawing from the penis completely and then just sinking down enough to tantalize your lips.

- In one of the woman-on-top-positions, try leaning forward and back, thus changing the angle of the penis inside you.

- In a rear-entry position, ask your man to stay still while you take control. Experiment with short and long movements. Also try rotating your hips.

Of course, you can also take turns moving. First the woman moves, then the man moves. Or you can both pull apart a little and then push back together.

The basic positions

The very fact that you're reading this book suggests you're interested in trying lots of different positions. Good! The *Kama Sutra* doesn't so much define specific positions as provide the basic principles from which you can construct your own. So the number is really limited only by your own imagination. As Vatsyayana explains, there are times when, for example, you want the *yoni* to feel tight – if, perhaps, an erection is starting to wane. And there are times you want the *yoni* to feel open – if, perhaps, you want to continue intercourse for a long time.

But there's a lot more to it than that. The ancient Hindus were incredibly aware of the relationship between body and mind. Yoga had already been around for thousands of years and *maithuna* yoga was, basically, sex. Every position has its own energy and its own effect upon the mind. If, for example, you want to copy those paintings in which the man and woman seem to be enjoying a sort of contented, mystical ecstasy rather than a passionate frenzy, then you need to know the positions that can help induce that sort of state.

Once you know the principles, you can become a virtuoso in sex. As the *Kama Sutra* says, the actions and movements of sexual intercourse 'cannot be defined'.

Twelve great reasons for using different positions

1 Different energy – There are positions in which you feel very close and intimate with stimulation all over your bodies. In others, you're connected only at the genitals, isolating and concentrating the impact there.
2 Different psychology – Whoever is on top tends to have a feeling of 'dominance' while the other tends to feel 'submissive'. In some positions this can be quite extreme while in others the man and woman are more or less equal.
3 Different view – Some positions provide less visual stimulation whereas others carry a powerful erotic charge.

4 Different tightness – Some positions open the *yoni* while others close it.

5 Different depths – Some positions allow extremely deep penetration while others keep the *lingam* within the entrance to the *yoni*.

6 Different muscular tension – Some positions create more muscular tension than others. When excitement is boiling up too fast, switch to a position with little tension; when things are going too slowly switch to a position with high tension that opens and stretches the thighs, such as The Pyramid.

7 Different stimulation – Different positions stimulate different areas. For example, rear-entry positions make it easier to stimulate the G-spot with the *lingam*.

8 Variety – Don't make sex a routine. Introduce novelty.

9 Rest – Sometimes you simply need to rest muscles by switching to a different position.

10 Practicality – When a nice comfortable bed isn't available you may have to find an unusual solution.

11 Fun – Trying different positions is quite simply fun.

12 Tackling inhibition – When you've struggled and wriggled and stretched and groaned and laughed as you attempt the more difficult positions, you'll cast off your inhibitions.

As we've seen, many different translations of the *Kama Sutra* have been published over the years, some of which have stuck with Vatsyayana's text and some of which have mixed it up with later commentaries. All very confusing. And the situation hasn't been helped by Vatsyayana's use of two different sources, a man called Suvarnanabha and a whole group of people together known as 'the Babhravya', who sometimes used the same name to describe different positions. Even more confusing.

For this book I was intent on uncovering the real positions, and that's what I've done. If you're just looking for ideas for sexual positions it may not matter very much to you whether they're really in Vatsyayana's *Kama Sutra* or not, or whether they're correctly described or not, but I thinks it's important to know you're really doing it the *Kama Sutra* way, like the ancient Hindus of 2,000 years ago.

Are you ready? Here, then, are the *real* positions from the *Kama Sutra*. Get your kit off and get started. You'll find the positions become a little bit harder as they go on (we'll move onto the very hardest ones in the next chapter).

1 Clasping position (man on top)

Vatsyayana says 'the legs of both the male and the female are stretched straight out'.

It might seem rather disappointing that the *Kama Sutra* should include the most 'basic' and best-known position in the world. But, after all, the missionary position is popular precisely because it's so good. Vatsyayana could hardly exclude it.

Have a go

With the woman lying comfortably on her back and the man lying between her open thighs, supporting himself on his hands or elbows, it's intimate, allowing for kissing, talking, eye contact and a range of caresses. The man is slightly but not unduly dominant – which suits the psychology of most couples most of the time.

The drawback with the basic missionary is that movement is restricted. Vatsyayana's 'clasping position' can be improved by the addition of a nice, thick pillow under the woman's buttocks. Not only is her *yoni* now raised for some intensive cunnilingus but the man can, for example, arrange himself on one knee with the other leg out behind for a powerful and versatile pattern of thrusting. With the man's weight taken off her the woman is also more free to move.

2 Clasping position (lying side by side)

Vatsyayna says this is the same as the previous position but with the man lying on his left side and the woman lying on her right side.

Have a go

From the man-on-top version, simply roll onto your sides without disengaging. This is a nicely relaxed posture in which you can just do nothing for a while. When it's necessary to raise the temperature a little the man can make the occasional thrust. When it's necessary to raise the temperature a lot he can lift his partner's upper leg for a view of her genitals and thrust more vigorously. After one side you can ignore Vatsyayana's advice about the man always being on his left side, roll right over to the opposite side and do it all again.

---

3 Babhravya's pressing position

Vatsyayana sees this as a variation on either of the 'clasping positions'. Burton and Arbuthnot's translation says the woman 'presses her lover with her thighs'. Some modern writers have taken this to mean that she presses her lover's body, but I'm convinced it really means that she actually presses or squeezes his *lingam*.

Have a go

If I'm right, this means that the woman's legs are pressed together to create a feeling of tightness in the vagina. Some translations say the woman does it herself while at least one other says it's the man who pushes the woman's thighs together. In terms of effect it doesn't make much difference. It's not so much a position as a technique which can be used in a number of different postures. You can do it, for example, in the 'clasping position' (see above) the 'rising position' (see below) and several others.

---

4 Twining position

Burton and Arbuthnot translate Vatsyayana as writing that the woman 'places one of her thighs across the thigh of her lover'. But that would be so banal as to be hardly worth mentioning. I believe the correct interpretation is that the woman places one of her thighs across her other thigh. In other words, she's intensifying the squeeze created by 'Babhravya's pressing position'.

Have a go

Still in a clasping (missionary) position, the woman crosses her thighs. Both of you will be intensely aware of the *lingam* inside the *yoni*, but the man will have to be careful not to be squeezed out. Crossing the thighs is also possible in other positions, such as the 'rising position' (below).

---

5 The widely opened position

Vatsyayana says that this involves the woman lowering her head and raising her 'middle parts'.

Have a go

The woman lies with her head just slightly over the edge of the bed, opens her thighs and lifts her hips by placing her feet flat on the bed and pushing up. This opens the vagina, hence the title. It also causes a rush of blood to the head, which some women like. If you don't, then keep your head on the bed. As a more comfortable variation, but with less tension, a woman can support her hips on two or three pillows.

Compared with lying flat on the bed, this method of raising the *yoni* has two particular advantages. Firstly, the woman's vulva is far more easily accessible for cunnilingus. Secondly, the man, now squatting or kneeling instead of lying, can move freely and tantalize his partner with a range of techniques.

'Unguent'

Vatsyayana suggests that when a woman is in the 'widely opened position' it's a good opportunity to 'apply some unguent' or, as we'd call it nowadays, lubrication. We've already looked at the various kinds in Chapter 06.

However, if a man is using condoms he's not going to notice it. Try this as a way of enhancing male pleasure. While the condom is still rolled up, fill the 'teat' at the end with water-based lubricant, then put on the condom as usual. During intercourse the lubricant floods out from the tip of the condom to produce an intense sensation of wetness. Some men like it so much they wear a condom even if they have no reason to.

6 Babhravya's yawning position

Vatsyayana says the woman keeps her thighs 'suspended' and spread 'wide apart'.

Have a go

As the name suggests, while the woman lies on her back her legs are well-opened and held up half-way between the horizontal and the vertical. This is a position which sets up tremendous tension for the woman, as well as stretching the 'sex nerve' along the inside of the thighs. It can quickly lead to orgasm. But no woman could maintain this position for very long. When you get tired, rest your thighs on your partner's thighs (if he's in a kneeling position) or squeeze your legs against his waist.

7 The rising position

Vatsyayana says this is when 'the female raises both of her thighs straight up'.

Have a go

This is one of those positions that sounds perfectly straightforward but isn't. If a woman has both legs straight up in the air, and together, it's impossible for a man to penetrate without a little ingenuity. If you don't believe me, try it. As Yashodhara points out, the woman's *yoni* needs to be raised. The easiest way of achieving that is simply to put a couple of pillows under the woman's hips or, alternatively, from the 'clasping position', the man can kneel up, hauling his partner's legs up with him as he goes. Another idea is for the woman to lie with her vulva at the edge of the bed while the man stands. Yet another possibility is for the man to open his legs and encircle his partner with his feet by her head. A fifth solution is for the man to lie sideways to his partner, a position nowadays known as the T.

8 Suvarnanabha's yawning position

Vatsyayana says that this is when the woman 'raises both of her legs and places them on her lover's shoulders'.

Have a go

As Vatsyayana doesn't say where her lover is when she places her legs on his shoulders there are all kinds of possibilities. The most straightforward is that, from the 'clasping position' with the man kneeling, the woman bends her legs up and draws them back so as to be able to place them on the man's shoulders. The man will have to move his arms (one at a time so as not to lose his balance) to allow his partner's legs to pass. You could stay like this but things get even more exciting if, once the man's arms are around the back of the woman's legs, he can lean forwards, maintaining penetration and, by gently pushing her thighs with his arms, tilts her pelvis up. In other words, the woman is now lying on her back, as before, but with her knees more or less on her breasts and with her calves and feet sticking up in the air. He can follow the movement by rising into a squatting position, or squatting on one leg with the other out behind. She can place her arms behind her knees or even, if she's supple enough, hold her ankles with her hands. For a man this is very much a position of conquest. His partner is utterly vulnerable. For that reason some women may object to it but those that don't will enjoy the combination of deep penetration, strong pressure on the vulva and the exhibitionism of openly displaying their *yonis*. The erotic charge for the man may be increased by pushing the woman into the position and then penetrating. This allows the man to see her *yoni* utterly exposed before, as it were, taking possession of it, while the woman can, with satisfaction, see in his eyes the excitement she is creating.

9 Suvarnanabha's pressed position

Vatsyayana says the legs are 'contracted and thus held by the lover before his bosom'.

Have a go

This is an easier version of the 'position of Indrani' (see next chapter). The woman, on her back, brings her knees to her breasts and places her feet on the chest of her partner, who will be kneeling. It's possible to make an enjoyable game out of this position. By pushing on his chest the woman can hold her partner away, a signal for him to tantalize her by keeping his penis just at the entrance to her vagina. Or she can relax slightly, a signal for him to plunge all the way in.

10 Suvarnanabha's half-pressed position

Vatsyayana says one of the woman's legs is 'stretched out'.

Have a go

This is a variation on the preceding position in which the woman keeps one foot on her lover's chest while stretching her other leg out straight. It can make her feel a little more open and sexy.

11 Crab's position

Vatsyayana says this is 'when both the legs of the woman are contracted and placed on her stomach'.

> **Have a go**
>
> With the woman on her back and the man kneeling, the woman bends her knees, splays her thighs open a little and rests her feet on her partner's hips. Her legs are now, indeed, like a crab's retracted claws. It's a comfortable position for a woman and good for tantalizing the entrance to her *yoni* as well as her G-spot.

12 Lotus-like position

This is not the full lotus but, as Vatsyayana says, merely with the calves 'placed one upon the other'.

> **Have a go**
>
> The idea of anything to do with the lotus position sounds pretty daunting, but this is actually quite easy for most women. The woman, on her back, pulls her knees back towards her shoulders, crosses her legs at the ankles and brings her feet as close as possible to her upper thighs. Obviously, she has to keep her feet clear of her *yoni* and it helps at first if she takes hold of her feet with her hands. The man, kneeling, now penetrates, pushing against her feet with his stomach. It sounds uncomfortable but it isn't. Its advantage is that it opens the *yoni* quite erotically and is very Oriental.

13 Supported congress

Vatsyayana says this is 'when a man and a woman support themselves on each other's bodies, or on a wall or pillar, and thus while standing engage in congress'.

> **Have a go**
>
> The advantage of a standing position is that it's something you can do anywhere. Well, not *anywhere*, but you know what I mean. Vatsyayana didn't specify any particular way of going about things so let's take a look at the possibilities. Seldom will *lingam* and *yoni* meet up without some assistance. For a face-to-face encounter it's usually a question of raising the woman up. A pair of high heels are a modern and enjoyable solution. Another is to make love on the stairs where height problems are easily resolved. It helps bring the *yoni* into alignment if the woman lifts one foot off the ground and wraps her leg around her partner.

Or, if the man stands with his back near to a wall, the woman can put one foot on the wall.

Ancient carvings and paintings also show standing sex from behind. It sounds impossible without the woman bending over but it isn't. The secret is for the woman to lean a little forwards, placing one hand on a wall for support, and lift one of her legs backwards. The man takes hold of her calf and raises her leg sufficiently to swivel her *yoni* to the rear.

14 Congress of a cow

Vatsyayana says that this is when 'a woman stands on her hands and feet like a quadruped'.

Have a go

Although Vatsyayana recommends copying 'the different animals' this is the only rear-entry position he actually describes. And, in fact, as a rear-entry position it has little to recommend it except for female ejaculation (see Chapter 11). It's uncomfortable and the woman risks being pushed over. It works far better if the woman can place her hands on something higher than the ground for support, such as a chair or the side of the bed. However, its great advantage is that you can do it in places like the shower or out-of-doors without having to find any comfortable place to lie down.

In the next chapter we'll be trying to work out, among other things, exactly how all those other animals mentioned by Vatsyayana, such as dogs, goats, deer, tigers and elephants, actually do it.

Summary

- The *Kama Sutra* describes nine different ways a man can move during intercourse.
- Women 'should do in return the same actions'.
- There are at least 12 good reasons for using lots of different lovemaking positions.
- The 'clasping position' (man on top) is the world's favourite, but can be improved with a pillow or two under the woman's buttocks.

- From there you can just roll into the side-by-side variation of the clasping position.
- 'Babhravya's pressing position' isn't so much a posture as a technique for squeezing the *lingam*.
- The 'twining position' is a way of intensifying the squeeze.
- The 'widely opened position' is good for cunnilingus.
- 'Babhravya's yawning position' sets up a lot of tension in a woman's body, leading to rapid orgasm.
- The 'rising position' only works if the woman is raised up or if the man sits with his feet by his partner's head or lies sideways.
- 'Suvarnanabha's yawning position' is highly erotic.
- 'Suvarnanabha's pressed position' can be used as a love game.
- 'Suvarnanabha's half-pressed position' allows a woman to stretch sexily.
- The 'crab's position' is good for the entrance to the *yoni* and the G-spot.
- The 'Lotus-like position' sounds difficult but is easy and very Oriental.
- The 'supported congress' can be used anywhere.
- The 'congress of a cow' can be used in the shower.

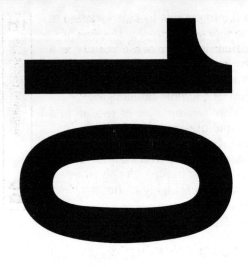

10 advanced positions

In this chapter you will learn:

- the most difficult positions from the *Kama Sutra*
- contortions inspired by ancient temple paintings and carvings
- ways of making love out of doors.

Even those embraces that are not mentioned in the Kama Shastra [Science of Love] should be practised at the time of sexual enjoyment, if they are in any way conducive to the increase of love or passion. The rules of the Shastra apply as long as the passion of man is middling, but when the wheel of love is once set in motion, there is then no Shastra and no order.

The *Kama Sutra*

So how did you get on with the easy positions in the last chapter? No problem? Good! Because in this chapter they're going to be getting a lot harder. If you haven't already done so, it could be a good idea to run through some of the warm-up exercises in Chapter 04.

Kama Sutra advanced positions

15 The position of Indrani

Indrani was the wife of the god Indra, so this ought to be a pretty special position – and it is. Vatsyayana says the woman 'places her thighs with her legs doubled on them upon her sides'.

Have a go

Some modern illustrated editions of the *Kama Sutra* show the woman with her thighs against her breasts, but this is not strictly correct. Vatsyayana says the position of Indrani is 'learned only by practice', so it has to be considerably more difficult than that. Early stone carvings show how it should be done. The woman lies on her back on the bed and pulls her knees back, not against her breasts but under her armpits, with her thighs as closely against her sides as possible and her calves closely against her thighs. Feet should be fairly near to the bed, not up in the air. You can help get into position by putting your arms around your thighs or, better still, taking hold of your feet with your hands. It's a position which has the advantage of displaying the *yoni* to the maximum while creating enormous muscular tension. However, it requires the sort of very open and mobile hip joints that only gymnasts would have. If you're not a gymnast, just do your best or stick to the easier 'Suvarnanabha's pressed position' (see previous chapter).

---

16 Splitting of a bamboo

Vatsyayana describes this as the woman alternately placing 'one of her legs on her lover's shoulder' and stretching the other out.

Have a go

This is one of those positions that burns a lot of calories. With the man kneeling and the woman on her back, the woman puts one ankle on her partner's shoulder and stretches the other leg straight out. She then switches, so that the leg that was up on the man's shoulder becomes the one to be stretched out. The best thing the man can do to help is keep his arms out of the way. The whole idea is to give a sort of 'chewing' motion to the vagina, so the leg positions need to be alternated fairly rapidly. It's tricky at first but, like everything, becomes easier with practice.

---

17 Fixing of a nail

Vatsyayana says this is when one of the woman's legs 'is placed on the head and the other is stretched out'.

Have a go

The question is, whose head is the woman's leg placed on? Some modern illustrated manuals show the woman placing her heel against the *man's* forehead. But Vatsyayana says the position is 'learned by practice only', which means this interpretation is far too easy. If we look at yoga positions, which go back as far as at least 3000 BCE in the Indus Valley, we can better understand what Vatsyayana intended. *Eka Pada Sirasana* is a pose in which the yogini places one of her feet *behind* her head, while *Dwipada Sirasana* requires *both* feet to be placed behind the head. Obviously this is the kind of thing Vatsyayana had in mind, with the aim of increasing the muscular tension and opening the *yoni*. Very few women will actually be able to get their feet as far as their heads but do your best to get one foot as close as possible.

---

18 Turning position

Vatsyayana describes this as the man turning round and enjoying the woman 'without leaving her'.

Have a go

This is a lot of fun (and the woman is going to have a go as well – see 'the top' below). The idea is for the man to begin in the missionary position and then, without disengaging, to slowly turn like the sail of a windmill so that he is sideways to his partner, then facing her feet, then sideways again and, finally, back in the missionary position. It helps to be well-endowed and to have a steel-like erection, otherwise it's all too easy to slip out.

19 Acting the part of a man

Vatsyayana says that a woman can act 'the part of a man' when her lover is tired, to satisfy his curiosity or to satisfy her own desire for novelty. In other words, she's on top. 'At such a time,' he wrote, 'with flowers in her hair hanging loose, and her smiles broken by hard breathings, she should press upon her lover's bosom with her own breasts; and, lowering her head frequently, she should do in return the same actions which he used to do.'

Have a go

Vatsyayana suggests that from the 'clasping position' and without disengaging, a woman should simply roll her lover sideways until she's on top. In other words, this is the inverted missionary. A woman could also start on top but the rolling over is a lot more fun – keep tightly hold of one another so the *lingam* doesn't slide out. However the woman gets on top, she can lie with her legs open or along those of her partner.

20 The top and the swing

According to Vatsyayana, this is when a woman is on top of a man and 'turns round like a wheel'.

Have a go

This, like the 'turning position', is something that can introduce a lot of fun into sex. While sitting on top of the man, the woman turns to face sideways, then towards the man's feet, then to face the other side, and finally returns to the face-to-face position once again. Vatsyayana suggests the man 'lifts up the middle part of his body'. In other words, he puts his feet and hands on the bed and pushes up. This is the kind of position men like to get women into so it's only fair if women turn the tables now and then. In fact, by thrusting up, the man is less likely to slip out, so it has a practical purpose. It sounds almost impossible but it isn't as long as the woman always keeps weight on one leg while turning. But if you do find it impossible, then, as illustrations show, the ancient Hindus always had cushions and couches at the ready. Much better to make use of such a prop. A couple, at least, of very plump cushions under the man's buttocks will give him the necessary support. Or he could lie, face up, across the sort of low stool or pouffe that was recommended in Chapter 05. For some women, the prominence given to the man's genitals can be very exciting. The woman needs to remember that her vagina is angled back up towards her spine at about 45 degrees so it'll help if she leans forwards a little when facing her partner's feet.

The 'swing' variation requires the women to swing her vagina around in all directions (in other words, 'churn') as she turns. This maintains excitement and helps the man to keep a strong erection.

21 Suspended congress

'When a man supports himself against a wall,' wrote Vatsyayana, 'and the woman, sitting on his hands joined together and held underneath her, throws her arms round his neck, and putting her thighs alongside his waist, moves herself by her feet, which are touching the wall against which the man is leaning, it is called the suspended congress.'

Have a go

This is the position that made the *Kama Sutra* famous. And, for once, Vatsyayana's description is completely clear. But how do you actually get started? The easiest thing is for the woman to lie on a bed or some other convenient piece of furniture with her vulva at the edge. The man then penetrates and, with the woman's arms around his neck, lifts her up with his hands under her buttocks. Now he can move over to the wall. It sounds athletic but with a large man and a small woman it isn't. On the other hand, with a small man and a large woman …

One translation suggests the woman should shift her weight from foot to foot against the wall. If you're a really athletic couple the woman can spread her legs out along the wall.

22 What happened to the elephant posture?

Surprisingly, aside from the 'congress of a cow', Vatsyayana doesn't describe any other rear-entry positions in detail, other than to recommend his readers to imitate 'the different kinds of beasts and birds' such as dogs, deer, wild boar, horses and elephants. Because of his mention of elephants, some modern commentators have assumed that the so-called 'elephant posture' from the much later *Ananga Ranga* is one of the postures he had in mind. It requires the woman to lie flat on her front and the man to lie on top, but as the ancient Hindus would have known perfectly well, no elephants ever do that. My theory is that the confusion has arisen because the position is suitable for the *hastini* or 'elephant woman' – a woman whose vagina has become slack due to childbirth. In other words, the position in the *Ananga Ranga* should be considered as the 'elephant-woman's posture' not the 'elephant posture'.

Have a go

When the woman is lying completely flat on her front it isn't possible for the man to enter, so she'll have to raise her hips for penetration. Once that's accomplished she can lie down flat again and the man lies on top, taking some of his weight on his arms. As a refinement, position a vibrator on the bed so it presses against the vulva.

Position 34 'riding a horse' is a better way of going about things – see below.

The mare's position and the pair of tongs

Some books about the *Kama Sutra* refer to two 'positions' known as the 'mare's position' and the 'pair of tongs'. In fact, they're not positions at all but *techniques* that can be used in almost any position, and they amount to more or less the same thing. There was a belief that a mare could actually 'catch' the stallion's penis by manipulating her vaginal lips. When a woman does the same it's therefore known as the 'mare's trap'. When the woman then 'sucks' the *lingam* inside herself and holds it there it's 'the tongs'.

Are these things really possible? Well, in fact, a woman can certainly contract her *yoni* around a man's *lingam* with considerable force and, by using a special technique, give her partner one of the most delightful experiences in sex. I'll be explaining how in the next chapter.

The contortions

If you've managed all the positions so far then you're obviously ready for the ultimate contortions. These are the unusual ones, the secret ones, the magic ones; the ones Vatsyayana had in mind when he wrote that 'when the wheel of love is once set in motion, there is then no Shastra and no order'.

These are what you might call *Kama Sutra* 'freestyle' positions. They're not actually in the *Kama Sutra* but inspired by it and taken from ancient Indian temple paintings and carvings in accordance with Vatsyayana's instruction that 'an ingenious person should multiply the kinds of congress'.

In actual fact, some of them aren't too difficult at all but, yes, there are others that really are contortions. Just keep practising the yoga and you'll be fine.

23 The pyramids

This is a position that makes you feel you've come straight out of the pages of the *Kama Sutra* because of the way it opens and stretches the body, and yet it's very easy to do. It's also one of the positions in which you both feel equal. The man kneels and either sits on or between his feet, whichever is most comfortable. He spreads his thighs and leans back a little, placing his hands on the ground behind him to help take the weight of his upper body. The woman now squats down onto her partner's *lingam* and, while sitting on his thighs, also leans back, just as he is doing, taking her weight on her arms. It's a position with a lot of subtle variations. You can both vary how much you open or close your thighs, to help control the sexual tension, and also vary how much you lean back so that you can be close and intimate or, at the other extreme, feel more in touch with the Divine Consciousness we discussed in Chapter 02.

24 Lotus embrace

This isn't a very difficult position but it is very Indian.

The man sits in the middle of the bed, with his legs crossed at the ankles and drawn up close to his body. If you can actually manage the half-lotus or even the lotus, all the better, but it isn't necessary. The woman lowers herself onto his *lingam* and sits on the platform made from his thighs and feet. To complete the posture, she places her legs around her partner's back and crosses her ankles.

It's a position in which you feel not just physically but also mentally intimate. You can chat. You can, as Vatsyayana says, 'talk suggestively of things'. You can share fantasies. You can drink. You can eat. You can co-ordinate breathing (perhaps while blowing in one another's ears).

It's not easy to move but you can both make churning motions and the man can stimulate his partner's clitoris with his fingers.

25 Lotus arch

In the 'lotus embrace' position, hold one another's wrists and lean right back until the tops of your heads touch the bed. The man's spine is curved back over his partner's crossed ankles while the woman's spine is naturally bent back to clear her partner's knees. This sets up tremendous energy through both of you.

26 Squatting embrace

This is similar to the 'lotus embrace' but the man has his legs out straight and the woman squats down onto his *lingam*, displaying her *yoni*, with her thighs well spread and her feet by his thighs. The woman can now move up and down on his *lingam*, keeping her vagina in perfect alignment for a truly ecstatic sensation. Her open thighs create a lot of muscular tension. He can rub her clitoris or he can take her buttocks in his hands, supporting her and guiding her movements, while his fingertips play with her labia and anus. If you want to make it more extreme, the woman can squat with her feet on her partner's thighs rather than on the bed beside his thighs – but not many women will be able to bring their *yonis* close enough to their partners' *lingams* in this variation.

27 The bench

This is a position with a fair amount of tension for both parties. The man, face up, rests only his head and shoulders on the bed while, with his knees bent, he has his feet on the floor. His abdomen and thighs therefore make a kind of bench which his partner straddles. It's a useful position because, when no bed is available, a man can just as easily support his shoulders on a chair, a pile of cushions or even a rock.

28 *Supta vajrasana*

The yoga position known as *supta vajrasana*, or the 'kneeling pose', provides the basis for this contortion. The woman kneels on the bed, her thighs comfortably apart, and gradually leans backwards until her head touches the bed. You'll probably need to do a few stretching exercises first. Your feet can be under your buttocks or to the sides, whichever you find most comfortable (or least uncomfortable). If you can't get right back, use a pillow or two for support. The position raises and opens the *yoni* and sets up a lot of tension. As is often the case, the man gets off lightly. He only has to adopt the standard 'missionary' position.

29 *Supta vajrasana* variation

The woman's position is similar to the basic *supta vajrasana* above, but the man's is different. The man sits on the bed with his legs straight and a little open. The woman now kneels astride his upper thighs and, as before, gradually leans backwards until the top of her head rests on the bed. She takes hold of her partner's ankles and he passes his arms under her back to help support her.

30 The bird

This is another of those positions that looks impressively Oriental and yet isn't difficult. The man sits comfortably on the bed with his ankles crossed. The woman sits down onto his *lingam* with her arms around his neck. The man then places his arms under her knees and around her back and in this way lifts her calves until they stick out horizontally like the wings of a bird. Since the woman can't take any of her weight on her feet penetration is extremely deep.

31 The jump of a tiger

Vatsyayana recommends a couple to emulate the 'jump of a tiger', although he doesn't actually explain what it is. This is one possible version.

Rather than stand on her feet as in the 'Congress of a cow', the woman gets on the bed on hands and knees. She can keep her legs close together, for a tighter sensation, or she can spread them widely to give her partner a full view of her. Her partner either stands with legs bent and well spread or kneels and enters from behind.

It's a rear-entry position that allows a man to see everything. If you're shy about that and have never done it before then try it first of all in the dark. There's also the likelihood of the vagina being pumped full of air, which then noisily escapes. But for the man, rear-entry can be powerfully stimulating visually as well as providing plenty of ways for him to excite his partner. He can hold her feet or hips. He can slap her buttocks, separate them, tantalize her anus and slide a finger inside. He can reach around and stroke her breasts and nipples or, reaching further down, her clitoris. He can lean forwards and nuzzle her ears and she can even turn her face to kiss. He can take hold of her hair and bite her neck which is, indeed, what animals do. And very exciting it can be (but not too hard).

For a completely different set of sensations the man can lean well back and you can then both concentrate on your own genital feelings.

As a variation, the woman can kneel on the floor and lean over the bed.

32 The congress of a deer

The woman, on her knees, bends forward and rests her face on a cushion. The position is subtly different from 'The jump of a tiger' because the vagina is tilted more upwards, creating a greater sense of openness. Again, the woman can keep her legs together or open them, as she and her partner desire.

33 The vertical splits

The idea of this contortion is that with both partners standing facing one another, the woman lifts one of her legs and places it on her partner's shoulder. I know, I know, only a ballerina could manage it. But what you can do is find something around the house you can just get your foot up onto. A sideboard, perhaps, or a shelf (preferably not one of those DIY jobs that could fall at any moment). Your partner now stands in front and you raise your leg and rest it on the support. Over time you may find you can get your leg higher and higher, which all goes to prove that sex really is good for you.

34 Riding a horse

The woman lays more or less flat on the bed, face down, and the man, on his knees, rides her, sitting on the saddle formed by the top of her thighs and the lower part of her buttocks. The easiest way into this position is for the woman to slowly lower herself down from Position 32 'the congress of a deer' because, once she is down, it's more difficult for the man to enter. Penetration isn't very deep but the head of the *lingam* is just inside the entrance of the *yoni*, pressing on the G-spot. This creates exquisite sensations for both, especially if the woman keeps her legs together (Babhravya's pressing technique – see above).

If the man keeps getting squeezed out then place a good, plump pillow under the woman's hips. You can both also generate interesting churning sensations and use your PC muscles to tantalize. While the *lingam* presses against the G-spot the woman can, at the same time, rub her clitoris against the pillow or, better still, against a vibrator placed on the pillow.

If you want to make it difficult, the woman can reach behind her to take hold of her own ankles. She then pulls her calves up and by opposing the muscles of her arms and legs curves her back into the shape of a bow. Because of the tension, this position can quickly lead to orgasm. But I prefer the version in which the woman bends one of her legs at the knee and uses her heel to massage her partner's buttocks and anus. A cunning move which, if the man isn't expecting it, will provide an extremely pleasant surprise.

35 The Seven Rishis

The old children's game of 'wheelbarrows' is also a sex position but hard to do and not particularly enjoyable. This is a sort of 'half-wheelbarrow', which is comfortable and fun. The 'Seven Rishis' (gurus) was the *Kama Sutra's* name for the stars of the Great Bear, which form the shape of a wheelbarrow.

To get into position, the woman stands by the bed and leans onto a nice soft pillow, laying her face sideways, with her forearms either side of her head, taking some weight. Her partner enters her from behind and then, while she keeps one leg on the floor, she raises her other leg so her partner can catch hold of her ankle and hold her leg up. It works best with a low bed so the woman has her head downwards. If your bed is too high, try using a couple of cushions on the floor instead.

36 The dog

For this one you both get on hands and knees and reverse up to one another. The man then swings his *lingam* right round between his legs as far as it will go and inserts it into the *yoni*. It needs a penis of at least average size and it works best with a taller man and a shorter woman, otherwise it's hard to get things aligned.

Adopting the position for rear-entry sex is something most women are used to but for heterosexual men it can be novel. A man experiences the same sort of 'open' sensation that women have. For the woman there's intense pressure on the G-spot from the penis because it's under tension. You can both reach between your legs to stimulate one another and yourselves or you can reach around behind and feel one another that way.

As a variation, it's possible to do the same manoeuvre standing, each of you bending well forwards from the waist.

A word of warning: it's better for the man not to ejaculate in this position as the penis is somewhat constricted.

37 The Khajurajo contortion

To end with, here is the most spectacular of all the postures, inspired by the erotic sculptures on the 1,000-year-old temples at Khajuraho in India, one of the wonders of the world. The woman is suspended upside down by her standing partner, with her head just off the ground, her arms around his lower legs and her own legs wide open.

But how to get into the position?

The easiest way is for the woman to bend over and place her head and hands on a nice pile of cushions on the floor. The height of the cushions is something you'll have to work out from experience. She then lifts one of her legs so her partner can take hold of it and support her. The next stage is for her partner to take her other leg, too, and penetrate her (not easy). She now gets a grip on her partner's calves with her hands while he shuffles away from the cushions.

And that's all there is to it!

Switching postures

It's fun to try moving smoothly from one position to another without disengaging. Thus, for example, you can roll from the man-on-top 'clasping position' to the side-by-side 'clasping position' and from there to one of the woman-on-top positions. A floor thickly-carpeted with rugs is excellent because it gives you the space to roll over and over. Otherwise, have the biggest bed you can afford and have room for. The key to it all is a powerful erection, otherwise the *lingam* is liable to slip out when you move.

But there may be times, on the other hand, that it's a good idea to disengage for a while. If a man is getting too excited, for example. After a break of, say, a minute you can resume in a new position.

Sex out of doors

Lots of Indian erotic paintings show couples making love out of doors, usually at night under the stars. It's a natural thing to do in a hot climate, especially if you happen to be the owner of a palace with a nice, secluded terrace. Not so easy, on the other hand, in a small back garden in the middle of a town.

In the West we're more likely to have the opportunity to make love out of doors when we're, say, walking in the countryside or swimming to an isolated cove or deserted island. At times like that, sex out of doors can be very special. If you're already doing something exciting that makes your body feel so alive, then sometimes you just have to have sex.

The problem is how to do it when you don't have a bed, a chair or even a cushion, and the ground is hard, uneven, stony or scratchy. Standing up is one solution. Another is for the woman to bend over and take hold of, say, a convenient rock or tree, while the man enters from behind. The 'lotus embrace' can work quite well because only the man's buttocks need to be in hard contact with the ground and they can be protected by throwing some clothes down. Or maybe you can find a convenient rock or tree stump to sit on. Other possibilities are 'the pyramids', 'the dog', 'the bench' and 'vertical splits'.

Garden swings

'In the garden,' says the *Kama Sutra*, 'there should be a whirling swing and a common swing.'

Swings are a common theme in ancient Indian erotica. In hot weather they're the ideal way of making love. If you have children you probably already have a swing in the garden. If not, you may have a swinging seat in the house. If not, get one. There are various ways of going about things. The easiest is for the woman to sit on the seat and for the man to stand or kneel, depending on height. It can be very languid.

Summary

- The 'position of Indrani' was named after the wife of the god Indra.
- The 'splitting of a bamboo' gives the *yoni* a 'chewing' motion.
- The 'fixing of a nail' requires a woman to get her foot close to her head.
- In 'the turning position', the man turns like the sail of a windmill.
- For 'acting the part of a man' the woman lays on top.
- If a woman swings while performing 'the turning position' it's easier for a man to maintain his erection.
- 'Suspended congress' is a spectacular way to make love.
- The 'elephant posture' never was in the *Kama Sutra*.
- The 'mare's position' and 'the pair of tongs' aren't positions but techniques.
- 'The pyramids' looks and feels impressive but is really quite easy.
- The 'lotus embrace' is great for talking and sharing food and drink.
- The 'lotus arch' circulates enormous energy.
- The 'squatting embrace' allows for a full range of stimulation.
- 'The bench' is great when there's a bed and great when there isn't.
- *'Supta vajrasana'* is extremely erotic.
- The *'supta vajrasana'* variation is the ultimate in *maithuna* yoga (sexual yoga).

- 'The bird' causes deep penetration.
- 'The jump of a tiger' brings out the animal in every couple.
- 'The congress of a deer' creates a feeling of openness for a woman.
- 'The vertical splits' is a great way to become more supple.
- 'Riding a horse' stimulates the G-spot.
- 'The Seven Rishis' is like the game of 'wheelbarrows' but much more fun.
- 'The dog' lets a man feel what it's like to be a woman.
- 'The Khajurajo contortion' is the most unusual position you'll ever try.
- Try to switch positions without disengaging.
- Standing positions are useful for making love out of doors.
- A garden swing can make a great sex accessory.

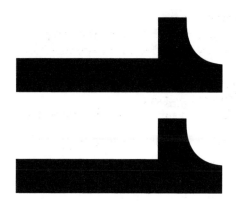

the *Kama Sutra* mysteries

In this chapter you will learn:
- how to stimulate the G-spot
- about *adhorata*
- about simultaneous orgasm.

At the first time of sexual union the passion of the male is intense, and his time is short, but in subsequent unions on the same day the reverse of this is the case. With the female, however, it is the contrary, for at the first time her passion is weak, and her time long, but on subsequent occasions on the same day her passion is intense and her time short, until her passion is satisfied.

The *Kama Sutra*

Several parts of the *Kama Sutra* remain mysterious. In every language one word can have several meanings and the Sanskrit in which the *Kama Sutra* was written is no different. The Vedas, possibly the earliest surviving texts in the world, were written in a form of Sanskrit that conceals secret meanings. Similarly, there are passages in the *Kama Sutra* that can be read in different ways. Did Vatsyayana know about the G-spot, for example? Did he know about female ejaculation? Those are some of the questions we'll be looking at in this chapter, together with the techniques.

The pair of tongs and the mare's trick

But first of all, a fabulous advanced technique about which there's no mystery at all. Vatsyayana says that when a woman (on top) holds the *lingam* in her *yoni*, draws it in, presses it, and keeps it thus in her for a long time, it's called 'the pair of tongs'. He also says that 'when the woman forcibly holds in her *yoni* the *lingam* after it is in', it's called the 'mare's trick'. One delightful technique, two names.

The *Kama Sutra* tells us it's 'learned by practice only, and is chiefly found among the women of the Andra country'.

What exactly were the women of Andra country doing? Well, the first thing they were doing was strengthening their PC muscles, exactly as described in Chapter 04. Once the muscles were strong enough they could then squeeze a *lingam* inside them, an extremely pleasant feeling for a man.

But there's an even better way of going about things. When the man thrusts in, the woman keeps the PC muscle relaxed. But as he starts to withdraw, she squeezes as hard as she can. There can't be many women who could actually stop a man pulling out. Rather, something better happens. The walls of the *yoni* are pressed tightly against the *lingam*, which is caressed along its entire length as the man slides back. At the same time, the *lingam* gives intense stimulation to the *yoni*. The result is an exquisitely electric charge for both of you. Keep it up as long as you can bear it.

Vatsyayana and the G-spot

Did Vatsyayana know about the G-spot? The translation of the *Kama Sutra* by Wendy Doniger and Sudhir Kakar (see 'Taking it further') says that when a man is moving inside the *yoni* and the woman's 'eyes roll when she feels him in certain spots', then those are the places on which to concentrate.

The *Kama Sutra* also says some *yonis* are like the tongue of a cow, which is a pretty good description of how the G-spot feels. So it would seem that Vatsyayana was at least aware that certain parts of the vagina are more sensitive than others, even if he wasn't specifically aware of how the G-spot functioned.

Nowadays we have a lot of research about the G-spot and know how to stimulate it with fingers or a dildo (which, as we've seen, the ancient Indians did have) as well as with the *lingam*.

Have a go: the G-spot

The G-Spot is named after the German researcher Ernst Gräfenberg although he, himself, never referred to it as a 'spot' because it's actually about the size of a thumbnail.

The G-spot is on the roof of the vagina and in the majority of women it's actually just inside the entrance. After pushing a finger through the resistance of the opening, the G-spot is the very next thing your finger will encounter on the roof. You'll know it at once because it'll feel slightly corrugated. This 'roughness' increases with sexual excitement so, if you can't find it, wait till things have hotted up a bit. Go beyond it and the vagina will feel incredibly smooth. And that's all there is to it. Smooth means too far, rough is right. (In a proportion of women, maybe a quarter to a third, the G-spot is further back.)

Now that you've found the G-spot, what can you do with it? Rubbing or pressing it will probably make a woman feel she needs to pee at first. Don't assume you're in the wrong place because there's no very pleasurable sensation. You're not. The G-spot takes time to get aroused and only then does the pleasure begin. It may help to stimulate the clitoris to get things going.

But not too much, because you want to keep the focus on the G-spot area.

Also remember that some women are very responsive to G-spot stimulation and some are less so. Everybody is made differently. But every woman can increase the sensitivity of her G-spot over time simply by stimulating it regularly. It can take months for the full response to develop.

During intercourse certain positions and techniques are much better for G-spot stimulation than others. In almost any position use churning (see Chapter 09) to press the *lingam* against the roof of the *yoni*. A rear-entry position such as 'riding a horse' (see Chapter 10) automatically brings the G-spot and the *lingam* into contact.

Did Vatsyayana know about female ejaculation?

If Vatsyayana more or less knew about the G-spot, did he also know about female ejaculation?

Certainly Yashodhara was aware of female ejaculation, because in his commentary to the *Kama Sutra* he writes about water flowing from a woman as it flows from a broken pot. He also quotes a verse that says women have two kinds of 'melting'. First a woman becomes wet. This, as we now know, was the 'sweating' of the vaginal walls which begins within 10 to 30 seconds of arousal (longer in an older woman). But after that, he says, if she's then carried away by her 'sexual energy' so she 'ejaculates ... just like a man'. So that's pretty conclusive. But he was writing a thousand years after Vatsyayana.

Vatsyayana quotes Babhravya as saying that 'the semen of women continues to fall from the beginning of the sexual union to its end'. That would have been the first type of 'melting', that's to say, the sweating of the vaginal walls. But Vatsyayana gives it as his own opinion that 'the semen of the female falls in the same way as that of the male'. That could well have been recognition of female ejaculation.

So what exactly is female ejaculation?

The fluid that women can ejaculate is comparable to the prostatic fluid ejaculated by men when their prostate glands are

stimulated (see below). That's not surprising b
also have a prostate gland (sometimes also kno
glands), located just beyond the front wall of the v
that you stimulate when you press on the G-spoi
produced is expelled into the urethra, the tube thr
women pee. The urethra, of course, has its outlet jus
entrance to the vagina and just below the clitoris,
quantity of liquid would be almost indistinguisha om
lubricant coming from the vagina. Hence the confusion.

But some women claim to ejaculate large quantities of fluid. In
fact, anything up to a cupful. These are the women who are
most enthusiastic about the G-spot area. They soak the bed.
They say female ejaculation takes sex to new heights both for
them and for their partners. They say the physical sensations are
intense and the emotional sensations even stronger. But given
the small size of the female prostate, how could such large
quantities of liquid be possible?

Devotees of female ejaculation insist it isn't urine. But when
there's a large quantity of liquid it's difficult to see how it could
be anything other than urine, slightly altered by the release of
hormones during sex, and with the addition of prostatic fluid
from the female prostate. Somehow, massaging the G-spot area
probably releases the bladder sphincter, which would normally
be shut during sex, and thus lets the urine out.

In the end, it doesn't really matter where the fluid comes from.
It's just a question of what you (and your partner) enjoy. If it
makes your eyes roll, do it.

Have a go – female ejaculation

To learn how to ejaculate it's best for a woman to practise on her
own at first. You'll have to stimulate your G-spot area with finger
or dildo for quite a while, certainly far longer than you'd have to
stimulate your clitoris to reach orgasm. You'll know you're close
to the point, when the G-spot area is hard to the touch, it feels as
if you need to pee and you also feel close to orgasm. Build the
sensations to a peak by pushing repeatedly for a few moments,
as if you were peeing, while keeping your finger still in your
vagina. Then remove your finger and push again, exactly as if you
were pushing to urinate. If it doesn't work in a lying-down
position, try again standing up.

you've successfully ejaculated a few times during
turbation you're ready to move on to intercourse:

- Make sure the G-spot is aroused, using the G-spot techniques described above, before the *lingam* enters the *yoni*.
- Get into the 'riding a horse' position.
- If 'riding a horse' doesn't seem to be working, switch to the 'congress of a cow' which, although less comfortable, can be more effective for female ejaculation.
- The man should use the widest part of his glans to move backwards and forwards and round and round on the G-spot.
- When the woman thinks she's about to ejaculate she needs to *push* and that includes pushing out the *lingam*.

Adhorata

Alain Daniélou's translation of the *Kama Sutra* (see 'Taking it further') sparked a controversy about *adhorata* (anal sex). In the Burton and Arbuthnot translation, the *Kama Sutra* had little to say on the subject other than that it's something done by 'people in the Southern countries'. But Daniélou's interpretation of the chapter on 'women acting the part of a man' was very different from the orthodox one. He understood it to mean not merely women getting on top but women actually using dildos on their partners.

Have a go – stimulating the *payau*

If you don't already then, man or woman, learn to love your *payau* (anus). It's an undeniably erotic area because it's absolutely packed with nerve endings and, what's more, it's contractions are part of your orgasm (unless you're over the age of 50 or so when it usually stops contracting).

The first thing to do is explore the sensations of your own *payau* with a lubricated finger, *once you're already excited*. (If you're not excited you won't feel very much.) Try running your finger backwards and forwards along the gully and then round and round the rim. You could also use a vibrator. If that feels nice, insert your finger into your *payau* as far as the first joint. If you enjoy it – and you certainly should – then you can ask your partner to do it to you while you're making love. You can also use your new techniques to pleasure him or her. Again, wait until your partner is already excited. It's quite likely the extra stimulation will cause rapid orgasm.

Have a go: *adhorata* (women)

Some women love *adhorata*, some give it a go to please their partners and some absolutely hate it. So don't make a big issue out of *adhorata* if your partner doesn't want to do it. It's her body and, frankly, it takes a lot of patience and skill (and masses of lubrication) to make anal sex pleasurable for her. Badly done it can hurt a lot.

From the point of view of hygiene, it's a very good idea for a man to dedicate one hand exclusively to anal stimulation and the other exclusively to clitoral/vaginal stimulation. Otherwise it's all too easy to get confused about which finger has been where. Anything that's been inserted into the anus (finger, sex toy, penis) must be thoroughly washed before anything else is done with it.

If you're both certain you want to try *adhorata*, first arouse one another. The woman then adopts the position 'the jump of a tiger' and the man proceeds as follows:

- Kneeling, slide your *lingam* into her *yoni*.
- During intercourse, play with her *payau* using a lubricated finger of your 'dedicated' hand (fingernail well trimmed).
- Once the *payau* is a little relaxed, gently push a lubricated finger in and out a short way. With your finger, you'll be able to feel your *lingam* inside her *yoni*, which is very exciting.
- After a while, switch to a specially designed anal vibrator if you have one. This in itself can be heavenly for both of you because the vibrations will be transferred to the *yoni* and *lingam*. Some couples climax at this point and don't proceed further.
- Once the *payau* is fully relaxed by all this attention, withdraw from the *yoni*, lubricate your *lingam* and insert a little way.
- Check that your partner is happy.
- Keep up the sexual excitement by playing with her clitoris (using the 'other' hand).
- Don't rush.
- If necessary, withdraw from the *payau*, apply more lubricant and re-insert.
- Again, check that she's happy.
- If not, withdraw and play with her again using the vibrator, your thumb or two fingers (and masses of lubrication).
- Re-insert.

Have a go: *adhorata* (men)

If, as a woman, you want to take things further in the way that Daniélou envisaged you'll need a 'strap-on'. That's a vibrator or dildo that's attached to a harness, as described in Chapter 08. Such dildos existed in Vatsyayana's time. Thus equipped, you have, in effect, an artificial penis. Quite a lot of women find the thrusting movement comes very naturally to them and enjoy the experience of reversing roles. Of course, it can't give you, as a woman, any direct pleasure, but if you choose one of the more sophisticated models you can get a built-in clitoral vibrator as well. With these designs, both of you can be stimulated while you're thrusting away.

As for your partner, he can adopt almost any of the postures for women described in this book. The Daniélou interpretation of Vatsyayana envisages the man lying on his back with the woman on top. But he could equally get on all fours or himself sink down onto his partner's '*lingam*' while she lays on her back.

If the idea of playing the part of a man so literally is too much for you, you could instead use a hand-held dildo or vibrator on your partner. One way of blowing his mind in a man-on-top position is to reach around and (if your arms are long enough) slide a well-lubricated anal vibrator into him.

There's really no need to feel apprehensive about the idea of *adhorata*. Just don't penetrate very deeply (say about two and a half to five centimetres) and there won't be any problem. The *payau*, rather than the rectum, is where all the nerve endings are, anyway, and the sensation of the muscle being opened and stimulated can be quite thrilling.

The only real reason to penetrate a man more deeply is to stimulate a special place deep inside known as the prostate gland.

The prostate gland is a vital part of the male sexual apparatus. One of its roles is to contribute prostatic fluid to the semen and the more it can be encouraged to produce, the longer ejaculation can continue. What's more, its contractions contribute to the pleasurable feelings of orgasm. So the prostate is one of the keys to great sex.

The prostate encircles the urethra, like a tiny doughnut, well inside the body just below the bladder and immediately adjacent to the rectum. At first sight, then, deep anal penetration would seem to be the only way to get at it. But, in fact, there are three indirect methods as well.

Have a go: the prostate gland

The first indirect method is to push hard on the perineum, slightly nearer to the *payau* than to the testicles. There's a sort of 'soft' area there. It's a spot where the finger can sink right in. However, this is probably the least effective way of stimulating the prostate. The second way is to employ the technique of sliding a lubricated finger in and out of the *payau* a short way. As we've just seen, this feels very nice. The finger doesn't reach the prostate but the stimulation it causes sort of 'spreads out'. The third method, and the easiest, is for the man to contract his PC muscle. The muscle needs to be quite strong so you may have to practise the exercises in Chapter 04 before you can manage it. As you contract the muscle you'll feel the sensation moving further and further inside. That's when the prostate is getting its massage. If you do this for a few minutes before having sex it's an easy way of guaranteeing a long ejaculation.

So much for the indirect methods. Now let's try locating the prostate directly:

- Insert a finger through the *payau* into the rectum, pad towards the navel, about 5.5cm – that's to say, up to the second joint or, in the case of small hands, the whole way.
- Press on the wall of the rectum in the direction of the navel. Don't curl your finger.
- You'll know if you're on the prostate because it feels quite distinct and is about the size of a grape (although it could be much larger in a man past 50).
- If you can't identify it as something quite separate from the surrounding tissue then you're not on it.

As a final test, play with yourself until you ejaculate (or ask your partner to play with you). The prostate will be felt to contract several times. Don't confuse the contractions with the pulsation of the blood vessel there. You'll know the difference by the fact that the blood keeps on pumping once the ejaculation is over, although less forcefully, whereas the prostate doesn't.

If you prefer, you can use a vibrator on the prostate gland, preferably one specially designed for the purpose.

Water games

Suvarnanabha, one of the sources Vatsyayana drew on, wrote that 'the different ways of lying down, sitting and standing should be practised in water because it is easy to do so therein'. Obviously the ancient Indians of Suvarnanabha's time must have invented the snorkel if not the aqualung! Vatsyayana took a rather ambiguous view. On the one hand he was rather worried that sex in water was 'prohibited by the religious law' (quite possibly a sensible measure wherever safe drinking water was in short supply). On the other hand he obviously thought it would be fun to imitate the elephants' water games (apparently they were said to orgasm almost immediately in water).

Certainly, water can add a whole new dimension to sex. In the garden in summer a well-aimed hose can be a good way of creating the wet T-shirt look as well as getting someone to take their kit off. A jet of water is also excellent for masturbating. Sex in the bath can be languorous, sex in the shower exhilarating. And if on a sunny day you should ever find a deserted beach then you may be more successful with the suspended congress in the sea than you ever were in the bedroom.

Apart from all that, some men find a cold shower after ejaculating serves as a pick-me-up for the *lingam* – and off they go again.

The long-timed man

Vatsyayana, as we saw in Chapter 09, says that if a man 'be long-timed the female loves him the more, but if he be short-timed she is dissatisfied with him'. Warming to his theme he goes on: 'In the beginning of coition the passion of the woman is middling, and she cannot bear the vigorous thrusts of her lover; but by degrees her passion increases.' If her partner fails to satisfy her, she 'shakes her hands, she does not let the man get up, feels dejected, bites the man, kicks him and continues to go on moving after the man has finished'.

So how can a man be sufficiently 'long-timed' to satisfy a woman and avoid getting kicked? One solution, according to the *Kama Sutra*, is to have sex two or three times during the day. A man may be 'short-timed' on the first occasion but he probably won't be the next time. Then there are ways of moving, as described in Chapter 09, that don't create much stimulation. And, as we've seen, there were aphrodisiacs which, it was claimed, enabled a man to 'enjoy innumerable women'.

But there is a simple technique for becoming 'long-timed' and it's known nowadays as stop/go. Basically, as soon as a man starts to feel himself becoming too excited, he ceases all movement and asks his partner to do the same. The best thing is for a man to practise on his own. Here's what to do:

• Masturbate as usual.
• As soon as you feel yourself getting excited, cease all stimulation and let your erection subside a little.
• Begin masturbating again and, this time, try to get slightly more excited than previously before letting your erection subside.
• Keep on like this, getting more and more excited by tiny degrees, until you do ejaculate.

Rather than having the vague aim of masturbating 'for as long as possible', many men find it easier to have a specific time target. In other words, if the longest you've ever managed before is, say, five minutes then set a target of, say, ten minutes. Put a clock where you can easily see it and make up your mind you won't ejaculate until the target time has elapsed. Once you've gained control on your own you can use exactly the same method during intercourse. Put a clock near the bed and keep an eye on it. Be determined not to come until the target time is up. If you achieve that, then next session extend the time again. Of course, you won't always make love by the clock. It's just to help you learn.

Multiple orgasms for men

Male continence and *Karezza*, which we met in Chapter 03, are basically styles of stop/go with a lot more 'stop' than 'go'. Eventually, the man 'stopped' completely without ejaculating.

Sex without ejaculation is arousing considerable interest again today. But whereas men following male continence and *Karezza* didn't orgasm at all, the modern method is for men to withhold ejaculation but still enjoy a form of orgasm.

If you don't already know about this, your first reaction may be that you don't believe it's possible. Your second might be, why would anybody want to do it anyway? The Victorians didn't have access to effective birth control but we do. So why bother?

In fact, this is the technique known as 'multiple orgasms' for men and the point is that multiple orgasms can both prolong and increase a man's enjoyment while, at the same time, introducing a mystical element into lovemaking, just as *Karezza* can.

If you're puzzled by this because you think orgasm and ejaculation are one and the same thing, then you're just making the same mistake that millions of others do. In fact, they are separate.

Ejaculation is the expulsion of semen. The word 'orgasm' covers the pleasurable contractions together with the sensation in the brain. 'Multiple orgasms' are not normal orgasms but what some sexologists call 'contractile-phase orgasms' or 'pelvic orgasms'. I prefer to call them 'partial orgasms', because that's what they are. Yet these partial orgasms can be exquisite. Once you get good at the technique, you'll find that each is more powerful than the previous one. Eventually you'll reach a state of ecstasy.

There are different ways of experiencing these partial orgasms without falling over into ejaculation. I'm going to describe the mental technique because I think it's the easiest and best. For a fuller account I suggest you refer to *Teach Yourself Great Sex*.

There first step is to refine the technique of stop/go during masturbation, as described above. Up until now you probably haven't been experiencing a partial orgasm. For that to happen, you need to improve that technique so you can get closer and closer to the point of no return. It's simple, but it's not easy because in order to experience orgasm without ejaculation you have to get very, very close indeed. Evolution has arranged things so the urge to ejaculate is extremely powerful. In order to 'beat' hundreds of thousands of years of programming you have to be resolute. You have to cease physical and mental stimulation instantly:

- Stop stroking your penis.
- Stop thrusting movements.
- Stop all muscle tension (for example, lower your legs if they're in the air).
- Stop breathing or, alternatively, pant (experiment to see what works best for you).
- Stop fantasizing (if you were).
- Stop looking at sexy images (if you were).

- Stop 'talking dirty' (if you were).
- Stop concentrating on the sensations.

In other words, you have to turn off like a light.

Don't be surprised if you don't experience much excitement from your first partial orgasm. It doesn't mean you've done anything 'wrong'. The second will be better. The third better still. Eventually, you'll experience sensations that'll be almost unbearably exquisite.

Once you've mastered the technique on your own you'll be ready to try with your partner. Explain carefully what you want to do because she's going to have to cease stimulation at the critical moment as well. It can help to divert attention from your genitals by taking your partner's tongue into your mouth and sucking it. It may sound crazy but it definitely works. It's not a technique in the *Kama Sutra* but it *is* Oriental.

Funnily enough, the greatest problem many couples have with this technique is not the man foregoing ejaculation for himself but the woman being disappointed. It can make a woman feel inadequate, in the same way that a man may feel inadequate if he fails to make his partner orgasm. Explain how great multiple orgasms make you feel so that she understands.

Simultaneous orgasm

Simultaneous orgasm is certainly one of the greatest experiences in sex. To enjoy the rapture at the same time is both exciting and uniting and it brings the active part of the session to a natural end. The *Kama Sutra* doesn't specifically talk about simultaneous orgasm but it does describe several techniques that will help you to achieve it.

If the woman has orgasms first, that's no problem. On the contrary, in a great sex session she should have several before her partner. But she can still have one final one – probably a 'bigger' one – at the same time as his. And she should. The real problem is if the man ejaculates before his partner has had even one orgasm. Unless he's unusually virile his erection will subside and the only way he can then continue to excite his partner is by using his tongue and fingers or a vibrator. But, quite frankly, his heart won't be in it any longer, because he'll already be succumbing to the hormones that'll make him feel unexcited and even sleepy.

If you want to co-ordinate final orgasms – and I recommend that you do – you need to discover ways of unleashing your orgasm and your partner's more or less at will. It helps a lot if the woman orgasms easily and the man has perfected good control (see 'The long-timed man' above).

The first thing is to agree that you *will* aim for simultaneous orgasms. Don't just leave it as a vague hope. You're going to have to co-operate and that requires a sort of plan that you'll both follow.

The next thing is to practise the techniques that are most likely to tip your partner over into orgasm. In other words, when you feel your own orgasm building, you need to be able to do something to your partner that will make him or her orgasm as well. Something powerful. Unfortunately, there's no technique that will make a man or woman come in a few seconds starting from zero. But there are physical techniques that will make most men and women come very rapidly if they're already quite excited:

- The most effective physical thing a woman can do to a man is push a finger a little way into his *payau*, as we saw above.
- The most effective physical thing a man can do to a woman is let her masturbate herself.

There are men who don't want their partners to masturbate during intercourse. Your man may feel that way. He may think that what *he's* doing should make you come, and if it doesn't then there must be something wrong with *you*. That's an attitude that needs straightening out right away.

The first step it to learn to masturbate together. If you haven't done so already, let him watch you masturbate. Once he's enjoyed that (which he will) you're on your way to introducing it into intercourse. Always do it in a positive way. Never criticize failures. Praise success. 'You make me feel so horny I've just got to touch my *yoni*.' That kind of thing. Explain that you're the only one who can manipulate your clitoris in order to come at precisely the right moment.

Then make it very clear that your own orgasm is building. You can simply say so, of course. That's a good start. But it will be much more effective if you communicate your excitement at the same time. Excitement is, well, exciting. It's catching. It will turn your partner on. The *Kama Sutra* is quite adamant on this. Make plenty of noise. Don't try to control your voice. Those initial groans tell your partner that you're beginning to get excited. Gasps indicate the approach of orgasm. Pants mean orgasm is being held off to build the excitement even higher. Words torn in half as if by the blast of a fierce wind mean that orgasm is beginning. Yells and screams mean that orgasm is underway. Holding the sound back represses the level of excitement. Letting the noises out builds it.

And talk dirty. The *Kama Sutra* says you should 'abuse' your partner. Exactly what you say is up to you. But lots of couples understand that the things they say during sex are a special case. Use the words you know your partner finds exciting. Try starting out with something like: 'You dirty little girl/boy ...', and then take it from there.

Summary

- The pair of tongs gives both of you – but men especially – the most exquisite sensations.
- Vatsyayana probably knew about the G-spot.
- Churning brings the *lingam* into contact with the G-spot.
- 'Riding a horse' is a good position for G-spot stimulation.
- Vatsyayana possibly knew about female ejaculation.
- Masturbation is the best way to learn female ejaculation.
- The 'congress of a cow' is a good position in which to try female ejaculation with a partner.
- The *Kama Sutra* mentions *adhorata* with women; some translators think it also refers to anal penetration of men by women.
- The *payau* (anus) is packed with nerve endings.
- A man's prostate gland can be stimulated via the *payau*, as well as in other ways, to create longer ejaculations.
- Elephants and people can enjoy sex in water.
- Women love 'long-timed' men; a way to become 'long-timed' is to practise stop/go.
- Men, as well as women, can experience multiple orgasms (although they're not quite the same as 'normal' orgasms).
- Simultaneous orgasm is one of the greatest experiences in sex.

12

watching the stars

In this chapter you will learn:
- what to do when intercourse is over
- how to massage your partner
- how to watch the gods making love.

At the end of the congress, the lovers ... should eat some betel leaves, and the citizen should apply with his own hand to the body of the woman some pure sandalwood ointment, or ointment of some other kind ... At this time, too, while the woman lies in his lap, with her face toward the moon, the citizen should show her the different planets, the morning star, the polar star, and the Seven Rishis, or Great Bear.

The *Kama Sutra*

In these few words, Vatsyayana beautifully captures the sense of intimacy and contentment that comes with making love. The ancient Hindus, as we've seen, liked ceremony and ritual. So it's not surprising that he should have been fairly particular about the way a couple should behave after sex. The complete list is as follows.

- The couple should wash separately.
- The couple should chew betel leaves.
- The man should give the woman a massage.
- The couple should eat and drink together.
- The couple should dance and sing.
- The couple should tell one another stories.
- The couple should look at the stars.

But the first thing a couple should do is simply lay together in one another's arms. Women take much longer to come down from their sexual high than men do. Anything up to an hour, in fact. So don't spoil that after-sex glow by rushing off to get on with something else. Revel in those feelings of sensuousness and togetherness.

Washing

With the passion over, Vatsyayana's couple become rather modest, 'not looking at one another' and going separately to the 'wash room'. But, in fact, showering together can be a nice way to finish. Soap one another then cuddle as you stand together in the stream of water.

Betel

As we've seen, betel leaves on their own amount to little more than a mouthwash. In this context they were, perhaps, the equivalent of the post-coital cigarette of years gone by. But don't be tempted. Smoking significantly increases the risk of impotence for men and the risk of gum disease for both of you. Hardly conducive to *Kama Sutra*-style sex.

Massage

In Western culture, any massage would be given *before* sex. But you can see why Vatsyayana proposes a massage *after* sex. With all that biting, scratching and smacking, not to say its violent thrusts and awkward positions, a woman is going to *need* a massage.

The *Kama Sutra* recommends sandalwood, but any nicely scented oil, lotion or cream is fine. The most important thing is to make sure it's *warm*. If not, the man should rub it between his hands for a while before applying it.

The basic strokes are these:

- Flat hands – Run them up either side of the spine, along the shoulders and very lightly back down the sides to the buttocks to begin again. Then move them in little circles. Finally, put them together on the skin then slide them apart to gently stretch the skin and tissue.
- Raking – Make your hands into claws and gently rake over the area you've just massaged.
- Feathering – Follow raking with the same movements but much, much lighter.
- Kneading – Just like a baker, 'pass' the flesh of the shoulders, thighs and buttocks backwards and forwards between your hands.
- Thumbs – Rotate the pads of the thumbs in small circles on the muscles.
- Fists – Pummel the flesh gently but rapidly with the sides of your fists.
- Hacking – Pummel the flesh gently but rapidly with the sides of your hands.

There's an excellent way of ending the massage which involves building tension throughout the body then abruptly releasing it. At an agreed moment, you cease all touching and your partner takes several deep breaths then holds one breath and clenches every possible muscle for 10 seconds. It helps to raise the legs, arms and torso for maximum tension. Your partner then completely relaxes and breathes normally. The effect is enhanced if he or she wears an eye mask and if there's some dreamy music playing.

Food and drink

The *Kama Sutra* recommends that, after the massage, the couple should 'eat sweetmeats, or anything else, according to their liking, and may drink fresh juice, soup, gruel, extracts of meat, sherbet, the juice of mango fruits, the extract of the juice of the citron tree mixed with sugar, or anything that may be liked in different countries, and known to be sweet, soft and pure.'

So all those things you got ready in Chapter 05 and didn't eat beforehand can now be produced. Vatsyayana says the man should invite his partner to drink from a glass or cup 'held in his own hand'. Alternatively, this could be the moment to play the old game of interlinking arms to drink. The Doniger/Kakar translation says the man tastes each dish in turn, comments on it, then invites his partner to try it. Of course, in our culture, it's just as likely the woman will have prepared these things and offer them to the man. The important thing is that the sharing of food and drink should be done in an intimate way. There's nothing like eating from one another's fingers, or even lips, to enhance that sense of closeness. And, for some reason, it all tastes better as well.

Dancing and singing

Put on whatever music you like to dance to and dance. And if you can sing along then, according to the *Kama Sutra*, so much the better. But the best kind of music for this particular moment is something really smoochie. You're in love. So put the lights down low (or light some candles) and dance close. It could be Diana Krall's *Love Letters*, 10 CC's *I'm Not In Love*, Fred Astaire's *A Fine Romance,* Chet Baker's *My Funny Valentine,* Sarah Vaughan's *I'll Be Seeing You,* Jack Jones's *What Are You Doing The Rest Of Your Life*, Frank Sinatra's *Moon River* and plenty more. Anything really mushy.

Stories

Arbuthnot and Burton's translation of the *Kama Sutra* says there should be 'agreeable conversation'. But other translations say you should tell one another stories. A verse quoted by Vatsyayana suggests you talk about the way you felt when you first saw one another and how unhappy you feel whenever you're apart. The main thing, of course, is that you continue to say loving and passionate things to continue the romantic mood. Don't start talking about the broken dishwasher.

The moonlight

Many of the beautiful paintings based on the *Kama Sutra* show a couple out of doors at night under the stars. Vatsyayana is quite specific that you should go out into the garden or onto a terrace or balcony and the woman should lie with her head on the man's lap 'with her face toward the moon'.

If you're going to try to impress your partner with your knowledge of the night sky you'd better do a little homework first. A planisphere is a pretty useful device. Usually made out of a couple of flat plastic discs it's the sort of thing you can slip into a pocket, refer to when your partner isn't looking, and then confidently point out, say, the seven bright stars of what the ancient Indians called the 'Seven Rishis' (gurus) and we know as the Great Bear or Big Dipper. The planets are a bit more tricky because, although they have regular orbits round the sun, their movement doesn't tie in with the movement of the stars. In other words, they can't be shown on the planisphere. If you want to know where the planets are going to be on any particular night your best bet is to refer to a website (see 'Taking it further'). With the naked eye you should be able to see Venus and Mercury at dusk or dawn, somewhere close to the path followed by the sun. Jupiter and Saturn look yellow while Mars looks reddish. The other two planets, Uranus and Neptune, are invisible. (Don't forget, Pluto isn't considered a proper planet any more.)

On a clear night, the Milky Way looks just as mystical as you feel. Remember that in Hindu belief you're effectively watching the gods making love.

Summary

- Women take longer than men to come down from a sexual high.
- You should both try to maintain the glow as long as possible.
- A post-coital shower together is one way of doing this.
- A post-coital cigarette is a bad idea.
- After all the vigour of *Kama Sutra*-style sex, the man should give his partner a well-earned massage.
- Share food and drink in an intimate way, nibbling from one another's fingers or lips, for cxample.
- Put the lights down low and dance to something really mushy.
- Talk romantically – don't mention anything else.
- Finally, look at the stars together.

taking it further

Thus have I written in a few words these Aphorisms on Love, after reading the texts of ancient authors and following the ways of enjoyment mentioned in them. He who is acquainted with the true principles of this science pays regard to Dharma, Artha, Kama, and to his own experiences, as well as to the teachings of others, and does not act simply on the dictates of his own desire.

Vatsyayana's concluding remarks from the *Kama Sutra*

Further reading

Translations of the *Kama Sutra*

As we've seen, the *Kama Sutra* was written in Sanskrit, probably in the third or fourth centuries CE. The 1883 translation by Arbuthnot and Burton was the first in English, since when there have been several others. All of the versions detailed below are in print.

The Kamasutra of Vatsyayana, translated by Sir Richard Burton and F. F. Arbuthnot, various editions

This was the first translation into English, appearing in 1883 and reprinted in numerous editions ever since. It combines the aphorisms of Vatsyayana together with later commentaries in a seamless prose which, although now dated, is easy to read. Although always attributed to Burton and Arbuthnot the translation was, in fact, a team effort. Two Indian scholars, Bhagavanlal Indrajit and Shivaram Parshuram Bhide, first translated the Sanskrit into a modern Indian language. An Austro-Hungarian scholar, Edward Rehatsek, turned that into

English. Arbuthnot then corrected any mistakes and, finally, Burton polished it and added some commentary of his own. Burton was a Briton with personal experience of Indian sexual culture and his interpretation of the meaning is as good as any foreigner's could be. But, inevitably, the manner of translating the work distorted the meaning from time to time. Given that Arbuthnot and Burton were in fear of the Obscene Publications Act of 1857 it was a courageous effort.

The Complete Kama Sutra, translated by Alain Daniélou (1994), Park Street Press

Daniélou's *Kama Sutra* is particularly interesting for two reasons. Firstly, unlike the Arbuthnot/Burton version, it separates the aphorisms of Vatsyayana from the later commentaries which, in this case, are provided by Yashodhara's *Jayamangala* (also used by Arbuthnot/Burton) and Devadatta Shastri, whose own translation and commentary in Hindi was published in 1964. Secondly, Daniélou took every opportunity to interpret ambiguity in an unconventional way. Thus the chapter that Burton and Arbuthnot interpreted as referring to intercourse in 'woman on top' positions, Daniélou translated as referring to women penetrating men and other women with dildos.

A member of a prominent French family, Alain Daniélou (1907–94) spent 20 years in India studying music and philosophy. He was a pupil of Swami Karpatri, studied cosmology with Pandit Vijayanand Tripathi and learned to play the vina with Sri Sivendranath Basu. His translation comes directly from the Sanskrit and, taking that together with his deep immersion in Indian culture, a great deal of weight has to be attached to his version. But although it's good fun, and extremely interesting, his version is rejected by most scholars.

Daniélou became a Hindu and ultimately returned to Europe to promote a more positive view of the religion. His other works include *A Brief History of India, While the Gods Play, The Myths and Gods of India* and *Shiva and Dionysus*.

The Love Teachings of Kama Sutra, Indra Sinha (1997), Marlowe & Company

Indra Sinha's interpretation is exactly what everyone would be hoping the *Kama Sutra* would be like. His verses are voluptuous and redolent of incense and sandalwood ointment. But it's also the freest translation, without any indication of what comes from Vatsyayana, what comes from Yashodhara's commentary and what comes from other sources.

Vatsyayana Kamasutra, Wendy Doniger and Sudhir Kakar (2002), Oxford University Press

This is an excellent translation that preserves the form of Vatsyayana's original. That's to say, the verses he quoted or wrote are retained as poems while the aphorisms are given as prose. Excerpts from Yashodhara's *Jayamangala* commentary are given separately as footnotes. There are also additional comments from Devadatta Shastri's 1964 commentary in Hindi.

Wendy Doniger is the Mircea Eliade Distinguished Service Professor of the History of Religions at the University of Chicago and has translated several Sanskrit texts, including the *Rig Veda*. Sudhir Kakar is a psychoanalyst and a Senior Fellow at the Centre for the Study of World Religions at Harvard University.

If you're looking for an accurate and recent translation, this is the one to get.

Other books by Sir Richard Burton

Personal Narrative of a Pilgrimage to Al-Madinah and Mecca (1965), two volumes, Dover Publications Inc.

The Perfumed Garden, Sheikh Nefzaoui, translated by Sir Richard Burton (2005), Dodo Press

Arabian Nights: Tales from a Thousand and One Nights, translated by Sir Richard Burton (2001), Random House

Books about Sir Richard Burton

Sinde Revisited: A Journey in the Footsteps of Captain Sir Richard Francis Burton, Christophe Ondaatje (1996), HarperCollins

It was during his seven years in Sinde from 1842–49 that Burton acquired his first-hand, practical knowledge of Indian sexual customs. A fascinating account of the key years.

A Rage To Live: A Biography of Richard and Isabel Burton, Mary S. Lovell (1999), Abacus

Isabel Burton has been vilified for one of literature's greatest [ ] of vandalism. After Richard's death she burned many of his [ ]ers, including his draft for a new edition of *The Perfumed*

Garden by Sheikh Nefzaoui. This is the biography that restores a little balance, giving proper weight to the influence of Isabel on Burton's life and work and proving that, in fact, the act of 'vandalism' was far less substantial than previously thought.

The Life of Captain Sir Richard Burton, Isabel Burton (2002), University Press of the Pacific

Written by his wife, this is not the most objective appraisal of Burton but it is the most intimate.

The Devil Drives: A Life of Sir Richard Burton, Fawn Brodie (2003), Eland

Another excellent biography of a man who has attracted such enormous attention.

Further reading on sex

Brauer, A. and Brauer, D, (1990) *The ESO Ecstasy Program: Better, Safer Sexual Intimacy and Extended Orgasmic Response*, Warner Books

Chang, J. (1977) *The Tao of Love*, Wildwood House Ltd

Chia, M., Abrams, D. and Carton Abrams, R. MD (2000) *Multi-Orgasmic Couple*, Thorsons

Chia, M. and Abrams, D. (2001) *The Multi-Orgasmic Man*, Thorsons

Craze, R. (2002) *Teach Yourself Tantric Sex*, Teach Yourself

Craze, R. (2000) *The Pocket Book of Foreplay*, Hunter House Books

Craze, R. (2000) *The Pocket Book of Sexual Fantasies*, Hunter House Books

Freke, T. (1996) *Exotic Massage for Lovers*, Eddison Sadd Edition

Fromm, E. (1957) *The Art of Loving*, Thorsons

Gach, M.R. (1997) *Intimate Touch*, Piatkus

Goleman, D. (1996) *Emotional Intelligence,* Bloomsbury

Hite, S. (1981) *The Hite Report on Male Sexuality*, Ballantine Books

Hite, S. (1976) *The New Hite Report*, Hamlyn

Ladas, A., Whipple, B. and Perry, J. (1982) *The G-Spot and Other Discoveries about Human Sexuality*, Holt, Rineha and Winston

Masters, W. and Johnson, V. (1981) *Human Sexuality*, Little Brown

Masters, W. and Johnson, V. (1966 and 1980) *Human Sexual Response*, Little Brown

Riskin, M. and Banker-Riskin, A. (1997) *Simultaneous Orgasm*, Hunter House Books

Sevely, J. L. (1987) *Eve's Secrets: A New Theory of Female Sexuality*, Random House

Stanway, Dr A. (1991) *The Joy of Sexual Fantasy*, Headline

Sundahl, D. (2004) *Female Ejaculation & The G-Spot*, Fusion Press

Walsh, A. Ph.D. (1996) *The Science of Love*, Prometheus Books

Information and products on the internet

Online encyclopaedia

http://en.wikipedia.org

Free and generally reliable online encyclopaedia, including sex along with everything else, written and updated by anonymous internet users.

The *Kama Sutra*

www.sacred-texts.com

A wonderful and comprehensive site that brings together most of the world's sacred and not quite so sacred texts, including, along with the *Kama Sutra*, the *Ananga Ranga* and *The Perfumed Garden*.

Hinduism

www.atributetohinduism.com

A truly fascinating site that explores the many facets of Hindu belief and achievement. If you want to understand the culture that gave rise to the *Kama Sutra* this is a good place to begin.

Indian erotic art

www.kamat.com

A very individualistic introduction to the erotic paintings and sculptures in India's temples.

Indian history

www.fsmitha.com
www.sscnet.ucla.edu/southasia/History

Everything you need to know about the time Vatsyayana lived … and before … and after.

My secret life

www.my-secret-life.com

The full text of one of the most famous examples of Victorian pornography, originally in 11 volumes and written by 'Walter'. If you want to know what the Victorians (some of them, anyway) did and didn't know about sex you'll find out by reading this.

Karezza

www.reuniting.info
www.luckymojo.com

Karezza, as we've seen, was a Victorian way of making love without orgasm. It has some ideas in common with Indian eroticism.

Flowers and garlands

www.save-on-crafts.com
www.chinaberry.com
www.webindia123.com

Information and materials for making garlands using paper, silk and real flowers.

Henna

www.hennapage.com
www.hennacrazy.com
www.hennaspirit.com

All the information and materials you need to decorate your body with henna.

Body art

www.bodydeco.co.uk

If you don't want to use henna, you can obtain all kinds of other products on this site.

Incense

www.simplyincense.co.uk
www.incense-man.co.uk
www.holisticshop.co.uk
www.onevillage.org/aromatics.htm

For all your incense needs.

Indian music

www.amazon.com
www.amazon.co.uk

To start with, try *India – An Anthology of Indian Classical Music: A Tribute to Alan Daniélou,* Unesco, 1999. It's a three-CD set in tribute to a man who translated the *Kama Sutra* in the most daring and unconventional way.

Indian herbs and aphrodisiacs

www.consumerlab.com

An excellent site that tests all kinds of health products, not just aphrodisiacs. You can read a brief overview of the findings for free but if you want to see the detailed reports on efficacy as well as side-effects then you'll have to pay either an annual subscription or per report. It can be well worth it.

www.himalayahealthcare.com

Extremely useful and detailed site about Ayurvedic medicine and the plants and herbs that can be used for sex as well as for a range of health problems.

www.frlht.org.in

An encyclopaedia of India's medicinal plants; rather technical but informative.

Apadravyas (sex toys) and sex furniture

UK

www.passion8.com – a reliable UK supplier with a wide range of *apadravyas*, lingerie, lubricants and erotica.

www.coco-de-mer-shop.co.uk – the mailorder department of the elegant Covent Garden shop selling luxurious jade dildos, edible massage oils, body jewellery, whips and, in fact, everything for *Kama Sutra*-style sex.

www.sextoys.co.uk
www.bedroompleasures.co.uk
www.lovehoney.co.uk

USA

http://store.sextoys.sex-superstore.com
www.toyssexshop.com

Penis enlargement

www.thundersplace.com

Useful information about penis enlargement as well as a forum for those who've tried it.

The night sky

http://space.jpl.nasa.gov/

A simulation of the night sky from the Jet Propulsion Laboratory at the California Institute of Technology, it allows you to specify planets, other bodies and even satellites whose position you want to know. It's not as clear as it could be but it should be enough for you to impress your partner.

www.nineplanets.org/nineplanets.html

Since this site was set up, Pluto has been downgraded and the nine planets have become eight. Oh, well! A good site for the sort of background information you might like to throw in while your partner reclines on your lap.

www.skymaps.com

A site from which you can download maps of the night sky for various dates.

Massage courses

www.massagefree.com
www.tantra_sex.com/tantra.html

Contraception

UK

www.brook.org.uk
www.netdoctor.co.uk/sex
www.thesite.org
www.spired.com

USA

www.avert.org
www.choose-health.com
http://dmoz.org/health/reproductive_health/

Sex technique

www.bettydodson.com
www.ivillage.co.uk/relationships/sex.html
http://sexuality.about.com
www.sexuality.org
www.take-it-like-a-man.com

Sexual health

www.bupa.co.uk
www.cdc.gov/std/healthcomm/fact_sheets.htm
http://health.discovery.com
www.healthsquare.com
www.sexualwellness.org
www.womenshealthlondon.org.uk
www.youandaids.org

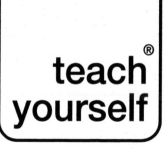

teach yourself ®

From Advanced Sudoku to Zulu, you'll find everything you need in the **teach yourself** range, in books, on CD and on DVD.

Visit **www.teachyourself.co.uk** for more details.

Advanced Sudoku and Kakuro
Afrikaans
Alexander Technique
Algebra
Ancient Greek
Applied Psychology
Arabic
Aromatherapy
Art History
Astrology
Astronomy
AutoCAD 2004
AutoCAD 2007
Ayurveda
Baby Massage and Yoga
Baby Signing
Baby Sleep
Bach Flower Remedies
Backgammon
Ballroom Dancing
Basic Accounting
Basic Computer Skills
Basic Mathematics
Beauty
Beekeeping
Beginner's Arabic Script
Beginner's Chinese Script
Beginner's Dutch
Beginner's French

Beginner's German
Beginner's Greek
Beginner's Greek Script
Beginner's Hindi
Beginner's Italian
Beginner's Japanese
Beginner's Japanese Script
Beginner's Latin
Beginner's Mandarin Chinese
Beginner's Portuguese
Beginner's Russian
Beginner's Russian Script
Beginner's Spanish
Beginner's Turkish
Beginner's Urdu Script
Bengali
Better Bridge
Better Chess
Better Driving
Better Handwriting
Biblical Hebrew
Biology
Birdwatching
Blogging
Body Language
Book Keeping
Brazilian Portuguese
Bridge
British Empire, The

British Monarchy from Henry VIII, The
Buddhism
Bulgarian
Business Chinese
Business French
Business Japanese
Business Plans
Business Spanish
Business Studies
Buying a Home in France
Buying a Home in Italy
Buying a Home in Portugal
Buying a Home in Spain
C++
Calculus
Calligraphy
Cantonese
Car Buying and Maintenance
Card Games
Catalan
Chess
Chi Kung
Chinese Medicine
Christianity
Classical Music
Coaching
Cold War, The
Collecting
Computing for the Over 50s
Consulting
Copywriting
Correct English
Counselling
Creative Writing
Cricket
Croatian
Crystal Healing
CVs
Czech
Danish
Decluttering
Desktop Publishing
Detox
Digital Home Movie Making
Digital Photography
Dog Training
Drawing
Dream Interpretation
Dutch
Dutch Conversation
Dutch Dictionary
Dutch Grammar
Eastern Philosophy
Electronics
English as a Foreign Language
English for International Business
English Grammar
English Grammar as a Foreign Language
English Vocabulary
Entrepreneurship
Estonian
Ethics
Excel 2003
Feng Shui
Film Making
Film Studies
Finance for Non-Financial Managers
Finnish
First World War, The
Fitness
Flash 8
Flash MX
Flexible Working
Flirting
Flower Arranging
Franchising
French
French Conversation
French Dictionary
French Grammar
French Phrasebook
French Starter Kit
French Verbs
French Vocabulary
Freud
Gaelic
Gardening

Genetics
Geology
German
German Conversation
German Grammar
German Phrasebook
German Verbs
German Vocabulary
Globalization
Go
Golf
Good Study Skills
Great Sex
Greek
Greek Conversation
Greek Phrasebook
Growing Your Business
Guitar
Gulf Arabic
Hand Reflexology
Hausa
Herbal Medicine
Hieroglyphics
Hindi
Hindi Conversation
Hinduism
History of Ireland, The
Home PC Maintenance and
    Networking
How to DJ
How to Run a Marathon
How to Win at Casino Games
How to Win at Horse Racing
How to Win at Online Gambling
How to Win at Poker
How to Write a Blockbuster
Human Anatomy & Physiology
Hungarian
Icelandic
Improve Your French
Improve Your German
Improve Your Italian
Improve Your Spanish
Improving Your Employability
Indian Head Massage

Indonesian
Instant French
Instant German
Instant Greek
Instant Italian
Instant Japanese
Instant Portuguese
Instant Russian
Instant Spanish
Internet, The
Irish
Irish Conversation
Irish Grammar
Islam
Italian
Italian Conversation
Italian Grammar
Italian Phrasebook
Italian Starter Kit
Italian Verbs
Italian Vocabulary
Japanese
Japanese Conversation
Java
JavaScript
Jazz
Jewellery Making
Judaism
Jung
Kama Sutra, The
Keeping Aquarium Fish
Keeping Pigs
Keeping Poultry
Keeping a Rabbit
Knitting
Korean
Latin
Latin American Spanish
Latin Dictionary
Latin Grammar
Latvian
Letter Writing Skills
Life at 50: For Men
Life at 50: For Women
Life Coaching

Linguistics
LINUX
Lithuanian
Magic
Mahjong
Malay
Managing Stress
Managing Your Own Career
Mandarin Chinese
Mandarin Chinese Conversation
Marketing
Marx
Massage
Mathematics
Meditation
Middle East Since 1945, The
Modern China
Modern Hebrew
Modern Persian
Mosaics
Music Theory
Mussolini's Italy
Nazi Germany
Negotiating
Nepali
New Testament Greek
NLP
Norwegian
Norwegian Conversation
Old English
One-Day French
One-Day French – the DVD
One-Day German
One-Day Greek
One-Day Italian
One-Day Portuguese
One-Day Spanish
One-Day Spanish – the DVD
Origami
Owning a Cat
Owning a Horse
Panjabi
PC Networking for Small
  Businesses
Personal Safety and Self

Defence
Philosophy
Philosophy of Mind
Philosophy of Religion
Photography
Photoshop
PHP with MySQL
Physics
Piano
Pilates
Planning Your Wedding
Polish
Polish Conversation
Politics
Portuguese
Portuguese Conversation
Portuguese Grammar
Portuguese Phrasebook
Postmodernism
Pottery
PowerPoint 2003
PR
Project Management
Psychology
Quick Fix French Grammar
Quick Fix German Grammar
Quick Fix Italian Grammar
Quick Fix Spanish Grammar
Quick Fix: Access 2002
Quick Fix: Excel 2000
Quick Fix: Excel 2002
Quick Fix: HTML
Quick Fix: Windows XP
Quick Fix: Word
Quilting
Recruitment
Reflexology
Reiki
Relaxation
Retaining Staff
Romanian
Running Your Own Business
Russian
Russian Conversation
Russian Grammar

Sage Line 50
Sanskrit
Screenwriting
Second World War, The
Serbian
Setting Up a Small Business
Shorthand Pitman 2000
Sikhism
Singing
Slovene
Small Business Accounting
Small Business Health Check
Songwriting
Spanish
Spanish Conversation
Spanish Dictionary
Spanish Grammar
Spanish Phrasebook
Spanish Starter Kit
Spanish Verbs
Spanish Vocabulary
Speaking On Special Occasions
Speed Reading
Stalin's Russia
Stand Up Comedy
Statistics
Stop Smoking
Sudoku
Swahili
Swahili Dictionary
Swedish
Swedish Conversation
Tagalog
Tai Chi
Tantric Sex
Tap Dancing
Teaching English as a Foreign
    Language
Teams & Team Working
Thai
Theatre
Time Management
Tracing Your Family History
Training
Travel Writing

Trigonometry
Turkish
Turkish Conversation
Twentieth Century USA
Typing
Ukrainian
Understanding Tax for Small
    Businesses
Understanding Terrorism
Urdu
Vietnamese
Visual Basic
Volcanoes
Watercolour Painting
Weight Control through Diet &
    Exercise
Welsh
Welsh Dictionary
Welsh Grammar
Wills & Probate
Windows XP
Wine Tasting
Winning at Job Interviews
Word 2003
World Cultures: China
World Cultures: England
World Cultures: Germany
World Cultures: Italy
World Cultures: Japan
World Cultures: Portugal
World Cultures: Russia
World Cultures: Spain
World Cultures: Wales
World Faiths
Writing Crime Fiction
Writing for Children
Writing for Magazines
Writing a Novel
Writing Poetry
Xhosa
Yiddish
Yoga
Zen
Zulu

great sex
paul jenner

- Do you want the best possible sex life?
- Would you like to enjoy sex at any age?
- Do you want both physical and emotional tips?

Whatever your age, background or fitness, **Great Sex** will give you everything you could want to enjoy a sex life that is not just exciting but totally fulfilling. From overcoming inhibitions to discovering your partner's desires and, of course, the latest, hottest practical techniques, this sensitive and enjoyable guidebook will kick-start your relationship both physically and emotionally.

Paul Jenner is a full time writer and journalist. Formerly a dealer in erotic art, he is the author of a dozen books and a regular contributor to television, newspapers and magazines.

tantric sex
richard craze

- Do you want to know more about tantric sex?
- Do you want practical advice and techniques?
- Do you want to deepen your spritual relationship?

If you've ever wondered what tantric sex is all about, this book demystifies an ancient practice. It draws on both the Kama Sutra and the latest sexual techniques to offer a complete guide to a tantric relationship. With practical assignments for men, women and couples, a guide to the latest 'toys' and plenty of further resources, **Tantric Sex** will enhance both your spiritual and physical relationship.

Richard Craze is an author and publisher of books on health, religion and a variety of related subjects.

teach yourself	**flirting** sam van rood

- Would you like to be confident with the opposite sex?
- Do you need advice on the dos and don'ts?
- Do you want to flirt at – and for – work?

Whether you are old or young, male or female, **Flirting** will give you everything you need to feel totally comfortable with the opposite sex. From pubs and clubs to the supermarket and the student scene, this practical guide offers case studies, exercises, top tips and even suggestions for how to flirt for professional as well as personal success. With an accompanying CD full of the author's coaching tips, this book will take your social life to a new high.

Sam van Rood is a qualified NLP coach who, as the 'date doctor' has helped hundreds of singles to relationship success through websites, television, radio, magazines and one-to-one coaching.

teach
yourself

life coaching
jeff archer

- Do you need your life overhauled?
- Would you like to be satisfied at work and home?
- Do you want strategies for long-term success?

If you've ever wanted to boost your confidence and set yourself new goals, **Life Coaching** is for you. It gives you direct, friendly motivation to review your aims, challenge your negative beliefs, and achieve fulfilment in all areas. It also provides checklists, case studies and all the practical resources you need to get where you want to be professionally, personally and financially.

Jeff Archer is a coach and director at Upgrade My Life, a life coaching consultancy that works with individuals and organizations helping them to reach peak performance. He is a regular contributor to a wide range of national media, newspapers and magazines.

teach yourself

massage
denise whichello brown

- Are you interested in the benefits of massage?
- Do you want to learn a variety of techniques?
- Would you like to know about oils and different kinds of massage?

Massage introduces both the practical skills and the spiritual principles behind an ancient and highly influential practice. Follow this illustrated guide to learn about everything from stress relief, treating sports injuries and self-massage, to using massage in relationships and while pregnant. This new edition includes even more practical advice and medical background, as well as fully updated resources and information.

Denise Whichello Brown is a highly acclaimed practitioner, lecturer and author of international repute, with over 20 years' experience in complementary medicine.

| teach yourself | **yoga** |
| | mary stewart |

- Are you interested in the origins and history of yoga?
- Do you want to find out if yoga might be right for you?
- Would you like to make it part of your everyday life?

Yoga explains both the theory and practice of yoga. With clear, step-by-step illustrations it explains yoga breathing and meditation and shows you how to perform the poses, to promote flexibility and strength and relieve the stress of everyday living. Find out how this ancient system of meditation and exercise can transform your life!

Mary Stewart has been teaching yoga for over 30 years and is the author of five books on the subject.

pilates

matthew aldrich

- Would you like to know more about Pilates and its benefits?
- Are you interested in improving your fitness and toning up?
- Do you want to find out why Pilates is so popular?

Pilates is an easy-to-follow introduction for everybody who wants to know more about the origins, theory and practice of this popular technique. Packed with useful exercises suitable for both newcomers and those already practising, this guide will ensure you benefit from all the health advantages that Pilates offers. This new edition is fully updated with a comprehensive introduction to abdominal exercises and the latest classes and resources.

Matthew Aldrich has been teaching and working within the health industry for over 17 years. The aim of this book and his work is to help you to get the most out of your body and your life.

teach
yourself

relaxation
richard craze

- Do you want to learn how to release tension?
- Would you like to practise relaxation techniques?
- Do you want to boost your energy levels?

Relaxation introduces you to efficient physical and mental relaxation techniques, drawing on a variety of disciplines such as meditation, self-hypnosis, muscle relaxation and autogenic training. Fully updated with the latest information and resources, this new edition features a CD offering practical exercises, breathing techniques and 'quick' relation sessions.

Richard Craze is an author and publisher of books on health, religion and a variety of related subjects.